The Book about
STRETCHING

● *Other Foreign Editions of this Book:* ━━━━━━━━━━━━━━━━━━━━━

Swedish: *Boken om Stretching*, SölveBok, Ystad, 1982
German: *Das Buch vom Stretching*, Mosaik Verlag, München 1983
French: *Le Stretching du Sportif*, Edition Chiron, Paris 1983
Danish: *Stretching*, Borgen Forlag, Copenhagen 1983
Finnish: *Stretching-Venyttely*, Otva, Helsinki 1983
Dutch: *Stretching*, Uitgeverij Elmar, Rjiswijk 1983

● *Under Production:* ━━━━━━━━━━━━━━━━━━━━━━━━━━━━━

Chinese: The Commercial Press Ltd., Hong Kong 1985
Indonesian: Angkasa, Bandung 1985
Icelandish: Orn Og Prlygur HF, Reykjavik 1985

The Book about STRETCHING

By Sven-A. Sölveborn

Illustrations by Ronnie Nilsson

Japan Publications, Inc.

This is the English language edition of *Boken om Stretching* Published by SölveBok, Snårestad 8, 271 00 Ystad, Sweden

Published by JAPAN PUBLICATIONS, INC., Tokyo and New York

Distributors:
UNITED STATES: *Kodansha International/USA, Ltd., through Harper & Row, Publishers, Inc., 10 East 53rd Street, New York, New York 10022.* SOUTH AMERICA: *Harper & Row, Publishers, Inc., International Department.* CANADA: *Fitzhenry & Whiteside Ltd., 195 Allstate Parkway, Markham, Ontario L3R 4T8.* MEXICO AND CENTRAL AMERICA: *HARLA S. A. de C. V., Apartado 30–546, Mexico 4, D. F.* BRITISH ISLES: *International Book Distributors Ltd., 66 Wood Lane End, Hemel Hempstead, Herts HP2 4RG.* EUROPEAN CONTINENT: *Fleetbooks, S. A., c/o Feffer and Simons (Nederland) B. V., Rijnkade 170,1382 GT Weesp, The Netherlands.* AUSTRALIA AND NEW ZEALAND: *Bookwise International, 1 Jeanes Street, Beverley, South Australia 5007.* THE FAR EAST AND JAPAN: *Japan Publications Trading Co., Ltd., 1–2–1, Sarugaku-cho, Chiyoda-ku, Tokyo 101.*

First edition: September 1985

LCCC No. 84–082450
ISBN 0–87040–621–3

Printed in U.S.A.

Foreword ────────────────────────

Because of the remarkably good results it produces, the new flexibility-training method called *Stretching* has already come to play a prominent part in sport-medicine, a rapidly growing branch of medical science. Unfortunately, however, since information about it has been spread through a circle of especially interested parties by means lectures, courses, scientific articles, and person-to-person contact, knowledge about it is sometimes distorted or false. And this threatens to put Stretching into disrepute.

As a sport-medicine physician, I take great satisfaction in welcoming the publication of this book, *The Book about Stretching*, which describes the various performances and advantages of this new method comprehensively and exhaustively.

The author, who is a physician, a top athlete, and a handball trainer, has assembled, in an exceptionally creditable way, virtually all available knowledge about stretching. Because of its completeness, its informative text, and its instructive illustrations, it is to be hoped that, both within and without the Swedish sports movement, this book, which has no counterpart in Europe, will reach the widest possible audience in the shortest possible time.

KRISTER WULFF

Ass. Professor of Orthopedic Surgery and Traumatology
University of Lund
Swedish Society of Sportsmedicine

Contents ━━━━━━━━━━━━━━━━

Basic Program for Different Types of Sports, 77

This is Stretching ———————

• A Simple, Effective Method to Improve Your Flexibility

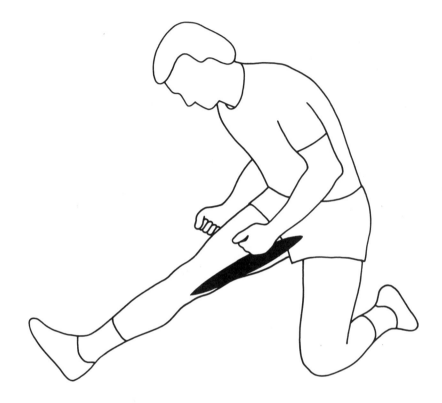

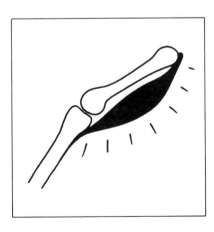

The best way to become familiar with stretching is to let the body experience how it feels. Try this typical exercise before you continue reading.

The basic principle is to first tighten the muscle, then relax it and then stretch it.

Place one knee on the floor and stretch the other leg straight out in front of you. Tighten the muscle in the back of the thigh by pressing the heel against the floor as hard as you can for 20 seconds.

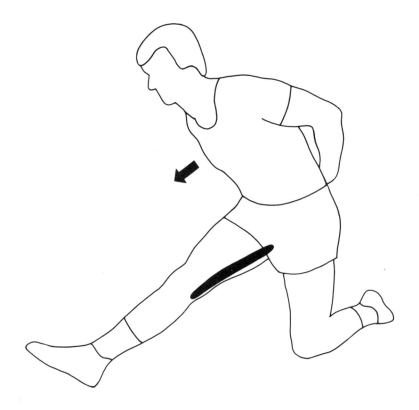

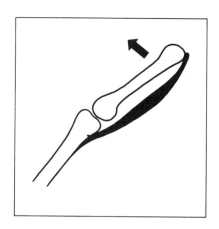

Relax two to three seconds. Keep your back straight and bend forward over the stretched out leg until you feel resistance. Stay in this position for 20 seconds.

This method in which the muscle is carefully stretched out is a prerequisite for increased agility and flexibility.

In stretching there is no *bouncing*. Bouncing stretches are of very doubtful value and can even be harmful.

Stretching: According to the Tighten-Relax-Stretch Method———

Stretching is the name of a new scientific method for simple, effective flexibility training.

Among athletes and those exercising for fitness, flexibility training has long been neglected. All attention has been focused upon conditioning (running/jogging) and building strength (weight lifting). However, to keep your body in the best possible shape all three are equally important: strength, conditioning and flexibility.

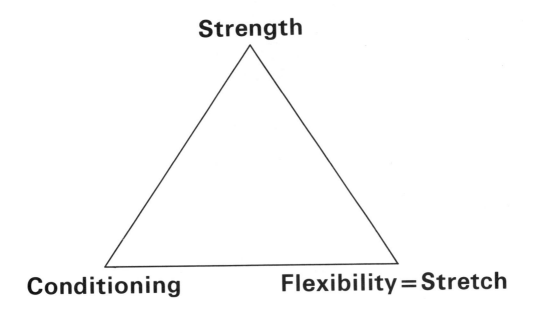

The stretching method totally replaces the conventional bounce-stretch exercises developed by the Swedish gymnast P.H. Ling—exercises that have turned out to be more or less ineffective and in many cases even harmful to the body. The term *stretching* consists of several procedures for stretching the muscles.

This is the basic principle of the stretching method recommended in this book.

TIGHTEN

1. Tighten the muscle or group of muscles with resistance and using as much force as possible without shortening the muscle. (Static/isometric muscle tension.) Keep the position for 10–30 seconds.

RELAX

2. Relax for 2–3 seconds.

STRETCH

3. Stretch out the muscle gently as far as you can and stay in this position for as long as you tightened the muscle (10–30 seconds).

This is the most gentle method of stretching, while at the same time giving a surprisingly fast and effective increase in flexibility.

The method has been used for a long time by some physical therapists and has during the last years been adopted by some athletic trainers and coaches.

The exercises included in this method are easy to learn and can be done year around without equipment.

They are also designed so that they are suitable for everyone: young and old, those out of shape and the physically fit, amateurs and professional athletes.

Some of the exercises can more easily be done with a partner. (See the List of Exercises further on in the book.) Others are made easier using a ball or gym equipment. However, there are exercises requireing no equipment for every group of muscles listed in the book.

Stretching exercises should be part of all training programs, both during warm up and during relaxation after a work-out. Since these smooth, harmonic exercises also contribute to psychological relaxation, the flexibility training becomes even more effective.

What is unique about stretching is that it also has proven to be helpful in preventing injuries. There is a definite correlation between tight shortened muscles and the origin of injuries. When stretching is done according to the tighten-relax-stretch method, the risk of injuries—sprains, strains and inflammation—in muscles and tendons is reduced.

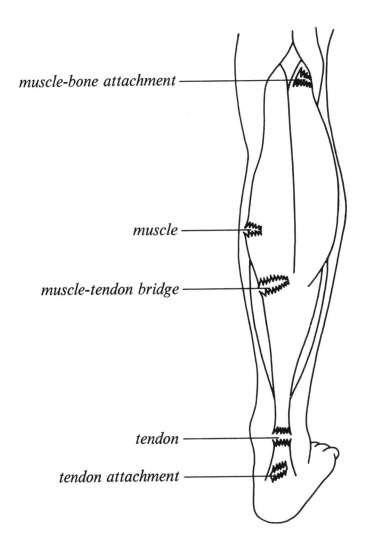

The principal areas where muscle tears can be avoided by stretching are muscle-bone attachment, muscle, muscle-tendon bridge, tendon and tendon attachment.

In addition, it is now known that stretching prevents decline and atrophy of the muscles which would normally occur because of inactivity, i.e., too much sitting or being restricted by a cast.

Some Important Words about Flexibility Training

There are three important words in the new flexibility training.

The first is **Stretch.**

When you stretch, you are starting with the muscle in an extended resting position. Then it is passively stretched a little bit further. The stretch is created when you keep the muscle in the extended position for some period of time (in our case 10–30 seconds).

The word bouncing (bouncing stretch) does not belong in our stretching vocabulary.

That is the old, incorrect method where you are extending as far as possible and then quickly returning. Exercises such as these can be harmful. Do not bounce!

The second word is **Flexibility**. It indicates the range of movement of the joints. (For example, the angle between how far back and how far forward you can move your foot.)

The third word, **Agility** is not the same as flexibility. Agility is the result of the nerves and the muscles working together, in other words what flexibility, muscle strength and coordination achieve together.

The ABC of Stretching

The Basic Principles

- Warm up and increase your blood circulation by jogging a little over a ½ mile. Include side-steps, jumping jacks and war-dance during the jogging. An alternative to this warm-up: Skip rope or do jumping jacks. Keep going 5–10 minutes.
- Tighten the muscle as much as possible without moving for 10–30 seconds.
- Relax totally for 2–3 seconds.
- Stretch gently as far as you can without feeling pain, and stay there for 10–30 seconds.
- Think on the muscle you are stretching and "feel" the stretch.
- Breathe calmly and rhythmically the whole time. Do not hold your breath.
- Keep the rest of the body in a comfortable position. The best effect of stretching is achieved when you are relaxed.

- Do stretching exercises for
  - —Chest muscles.   Exercise 2 (or 4)
  - —Back and neck.   Exercise 46
  - —Groin muscles.   Exercise 31
  - —Calves.   Exercise 39
  - —Front thigh.   Exercise 20
  - —Front lower leg. Exercise 43
  - —Hamstrings.   Exercise 22
  - —Hip-benders.   Exercise 36
- Work out on your own. If you have a partner, don't compare how far you can reach. You don't compete in stretching.
- Work out on a regular basis. At least three work-outs per week are necessary to ensure good results, but it won't hurt you to do stretching every day.
- If you are exercising some other way for strength, stamina or specific practice of a sport, you should include stretching in your current routine in order to maintain or improve your flexibility and to prevent injuries.
- Preferably, put the main stretching program after other exercises (especially strength training) during the so called "down training" ("cool-down" or "warm-down") portion, doing three consecutive sets of the exercises selected for each group of muscles. At the start of your training program, it would then be adequate to do one set of stretches for each of the specific muscles.

Some Tips

- If you want to increase the intensity of your training program you can do this: Use the furthest position reached in the first stretch as the starting point for a repetition of the same exercise with a new tightening of the muscle and then another stretch.
- After stretching a particular group of muscles you should also stretch the counteracting muscles (the antagonists).
- Stretch the front muscles of the thighs before stretching the hamstrings. This tends to yield better results.
- If you are tighter on one side than the other, always start with the "worst" side. You almost automatically spend more time on the side you start with.
- If the back of one leg, especially the thigh, is tighter than the other, or if you have or have had trouble with your lower back, do not bend and stretch both legs at the same time. Use exercises stretching one leg at a time.
- Be "back conscious"! Always keep your head in a straight line with your back.
- If a muscle feels extra tight, it is often advantageous to stretch the counteracting muscle first.
- When you stretch standing on your knee(s), the toes should always point straight back. If you put weight on the inside of the foot, the knee will get incorrect pressure.

- Refrain from doing your stretching program if you are injured or have pain in muscles, joints or tendons. If you have recently had an operation you should contact your doctor prior to starting your stretching exercises.
- The drawings in the exercise section show different positions for stretching. They are not intended to show how far you should stretch.
- Start and finish the stretch both smoothly and carefully.
- Finally: Don't bounce in the furthest stretch position.

Conditioning ————————————————————

Combine the stretching exercises with a conditioning program. Here are some simple alternatives for a basic program.

1. Exercising to build **stamina**.
    Run 2 miles.
    > OR
    Run 15–15 intervals, i.e., 15 seconds of running followed by 15 seconds of rest for 7–10 minutes.
    > OR
    Run 70–20 intervals, i.e., 70 seconds of running followed by 20 seconds of rest. Repeat 10–12 times.

2. Exercising to build **speed**.
    Sprint 30–45 seconds at maximum speed followed by 60–90 seconds of rest. Repeat 5–10 times.
    > OR
    Sprint 50 meters full speed, rest 10 seconds. Repeat 10 times. The intensity can be increased by doing alternating side-steps, 3–4 each way, during the 10 second rest periods in between the sprints. You could vary the sprints by alternating 30 meters forwards with 20 meters backwards.

3. Start and finish the stretch both smoothly and carefully.

Traditional Bounce-Stretching Gymnastics and Other Unsuitable Exercises ────────────

The traditional bounce-stretching exercises developed from ideas of the Swedish gymnast P.H. Ling are not particularly good.

The method is based on stretching the muscle to the furthest possible point, then bouncing back and then stretching again.

Today we know that these bounce-stretching exercises (also called ballistic stretching) most often do not improve the muscle elasticity. Rather they create tighter muscles.*

The reason for this is that the rapid bounce-stretch releases a nerve reflex that signals the muscle to contract. This stretch-reflex is a protective mechanism that prevents the joint from getting hurt when a stretch is going too far. Every bounce-stretch activates the stretch reflex. Since the created muscle contraction works against the stretching movement, the muscle fibers are torn. When they heal, scar tissue is created which makes the muscle elasticity worse. The muscle becomes sore and stiff.

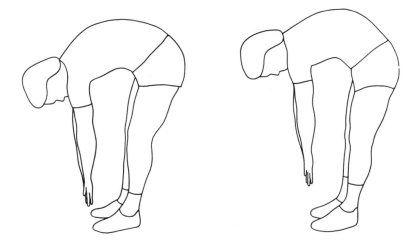

---

* You can very quickly demonstrate this for yourself. Just do this. Stand with your knees straight and bend forward with your hands stretching toward the floor. Bounce-stretch 4–5 times. Wait a few minutes. Bend forward again in the same manner. This time your hands are further from the floor than the first time.

There are some other common exercises that are unsuitable for other reasons.

Side-bends with a rocking motion are of no value. If they are performed with weights, they are actually harmful.

Head rotations have no positive effects.

Waist rotations are not particularly good. If you do them anyway, at least don't lean backwards during the exercise. Preferably the knees should be slightly bent when the weight is shifted from one leg to another.

Forceful back-bends backwards are not recommended.

Deep knee bends further than a 90 degree angle should not be done unless you are extremely fit.

Sit-ups should be done by lifting the head only up to no more than 10 inches off the ground. Then the stomach muscles work the most. Bend your knees to decrease the risk of back problems. Avoid sit-ups where you stretch the right hand to the left foot and vice versa if you have back problems.

If you are exercising your back muscles lying on your stomach ("Banana"), don't lift your chest and your legs at the same time. Diagnoal exercises (lifting right arm and left leg) are better.

Movement Exercises

Exercises that (without being bounce stretches) cover the whole or as much as possible of the joint's mobility range (and also similar strengthening exercises) are favorable from a flexibility point of view. Such dynamic, often rotating movements, can favorably be mixed in with the stretching program, which is more static in nature, to make the training session more varied and multi-faceted.

Examples of such exercises are:

- Running with high pull-ups of the knees.
- Running with the heels touching the buttocks.
- (Soft) leg kick, clapping hands under the thigh.
- Arm rotations, full circle (moderate pace) one or both arms at the same time preferably with accompanying movements in the knees.
- Arm pendulum movement forward-backward (both arms) with simultaneous knee-bends (*Maja*).
- Shoulder rotation with bent elbows, as big a circle as possible.
- Swim motion ("crawl") in slightly forward bent position.
- Groin rotation (with bent knee) standing on one leg.
- Lying down on your back, move legs from side to side, all the way down to the floor or in large circles.
- Leg shifts forward-backward from "push-up position" or side-to-side jumping from "knee bend position" without bouncing.

Muscles Overview (I) ——

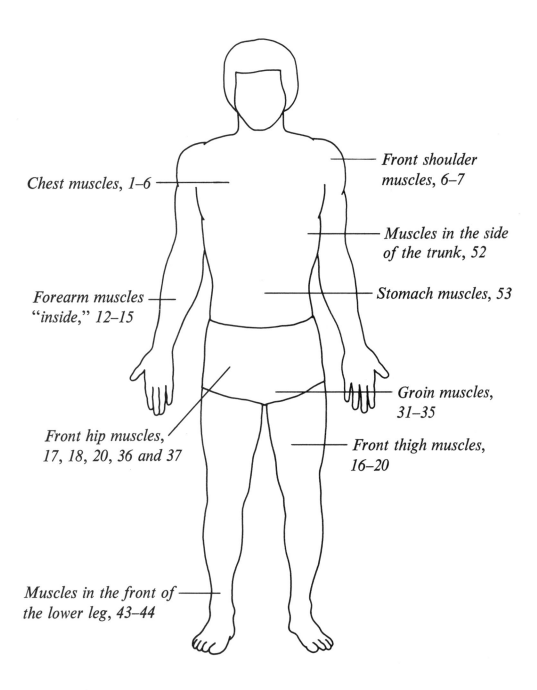

Chest muscles, 1–6 ——

Front shoulder
muscles, 6–7

Muscles in the side
of the trunk, 52

Forearm muscles ——
"inside," 12–15

Stomach muscles, 53

Groin muscles,
31–35

Front hip muscles,
17, 18, 20, 36 and 37

Front thigh muscles,
16–20

Muscles in the front of ——
the lower leg, 43–44

Muscles Overview (II)━━━━

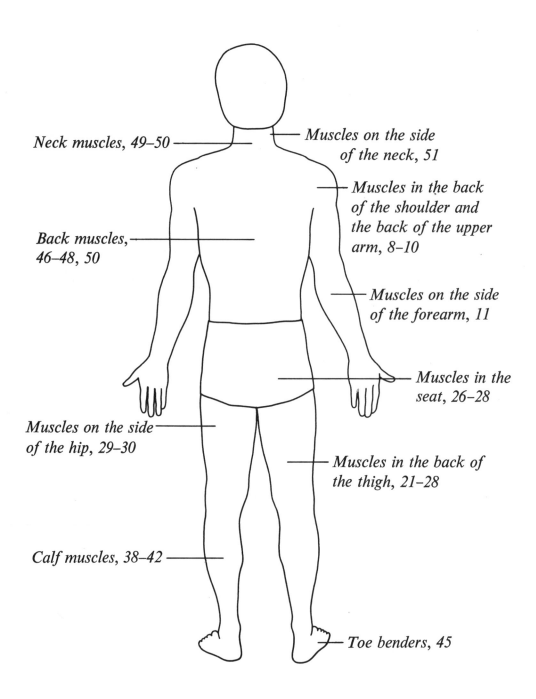

Neck muscles, 49–50

Muscles on the side
of the neck, 51

Muscles in the back
of the shoulder and
the back of the upper
arm, 8–10

Back muscles,
46–48, 50

Muscles on the side
of the forearm, 11

Muscles in the
seat, 26–28

Muscles on the side
of the hip, 29–30

Muscles in the back of
the thigh, 21–28

Calf muscles, 38–42

Toe benders, 45

Stretching
Chest 2, 4, 3, 9, 7, 5
Back & neck 46, 47, 49
Groin 31, 32
Calves 39, 41
Front Thigh 20, 17
Front Lower Leg 43
Hamstring 22, 23, 25
Hip flexors 36, 37, 30
Fore Arms 11, 13, 12

Movers of the Arm

ventralis/m. pectoralis major.

ted arm forward.

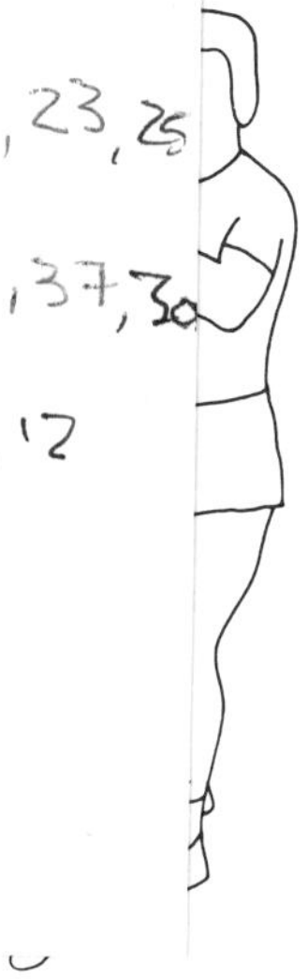

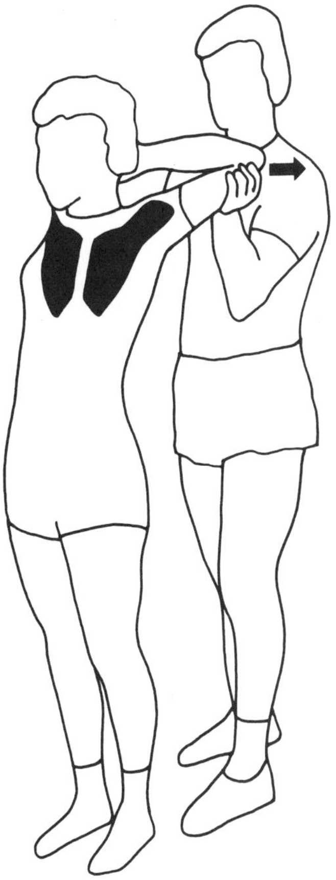

A. Tighten

Clasp your hands behind your neck and hold them against your head. Let your practice partner hold your elbows while you are pressing the elbows forward for approximately 20 seconds.

B. Stretch

Passive stretching by having your practice partner pull the elbows backwards and keeping the position for approximately 20 seconds.

2. Chest Muscles ———————————

M. pectoralis major & minor, m. coracobrachialis.

Function: *Moves the arm forward and inward in the shoulder joint and lowers and moves the shoulder forward.*

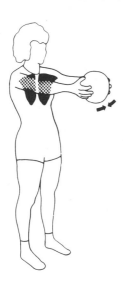

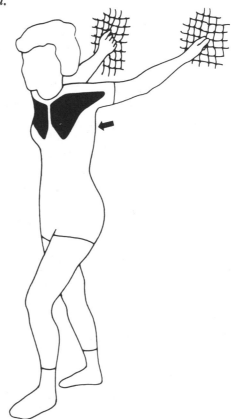

A. Tighten

Press (with or without a ball in between) your hands against each other as hard as possible with arms straight in front of your body for 20 seconds.

B. Stretch

Extend the arms backward-upward, preferably passively, and keep the position for 20 seconds by holding on to a net. The stretch can also be made with assistance of your practice partner holding on to your wrists.

Note: Both portions of this exercise can be made with you and your practice partner simultaneously. Stand with your backs against each other and grab each others hands with the arms lifted straight out on each side. First try to press the straightened arms away from each other through active muscle tightening. Then stretch the straightened arms by taking a small step away from each other without letting go of your hands.

3. Chest Muscles ─────────

M. pectoralis major.

Function: Moves the arm forward (and inward) in the shoulder joint.

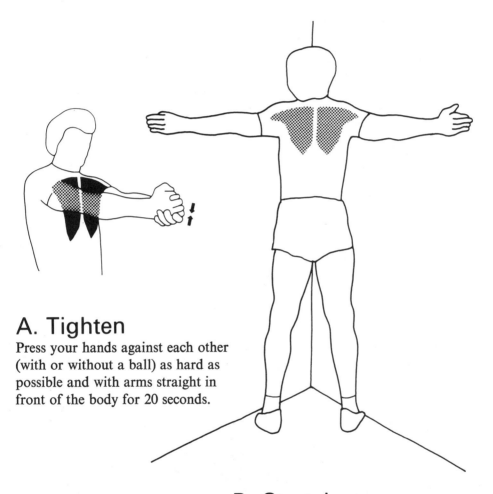

A. Tighten
Press your hands against each other (with or without a ball) as hard as possible and with arms straight in front of the body for 20 seconds.

B. Stretch
Stand in a corner of the room facing the corner. Put your hands (alternately your forearms) against the walls and let your body fall forward. Press inward so that you feel the tightening in the front of your rib cage for 20 seconds.

Note: The tightening portion can advantageously be done in the same position, in the corner, as the stretch. However, do not press in quite as far.

4. Chest Muscles ─────────────

M. pectoralis major, m. teres major.

Function: Move the arms forward and downward from a lifted position.

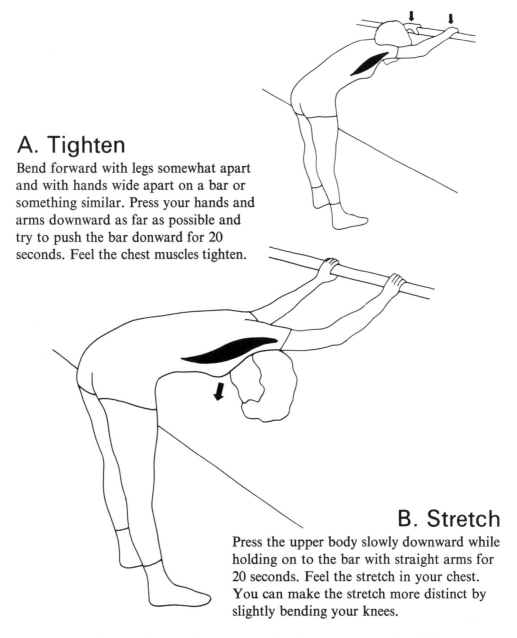

A. Tighten

Bend forward with legs somewhat apart
and with hands wide apart on a bar or
something similar. Press your hands and
arms downward as far as possible and
try to push the bar donward for 20
seconds. Feel the chest muscles tighten.

B. Stretch

Press the upper body slowly downward while
holding on to the bar with straight arms for
20 seconds. Feel the stretch in your chest.
You can make the stretch more distinct by
slightly bending your knees.

Note: By varying the distance between your hands you can practice different
parts of your chest muscles. By placing your hands at different heights you also
change the stretching area.

5.   The large Chest Muscles ——————

M. pectoralis major.

Function: *Moves the arm forward from the shoulder joint.*

B. Stretch

Keep your forearm in the same position
and maintain a stable base with your feet.
Turn your body out and forward so that
the chest is pushed forward as far as possible. Feel the tightening in your chest up
toward the front of your shoulder. Keep
the position for 20 seconds.

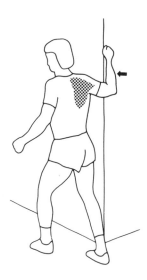

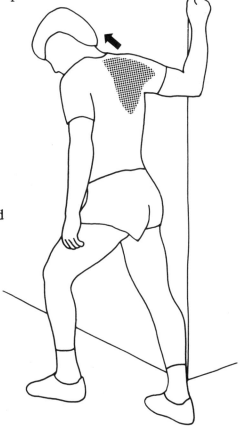

A. Tighten

Stand with your side against a door
frame and press your hand or your
forearm against the door frame as hard
as possible for 20 seconds.

Alternative: Instead of the door, you could hold on to a bar; standing with your
back against it, try to pull the bar out. Or the same thing with a net.

Note: By varying the arm positioning up and down, you can exercise different
parts of the chest muscles.

6. Front Shoulder Muscles

M. subscapularis, m. pectoralis major/pars clavicularis.

Function: Rotates the arm inward from the shoulder joint.

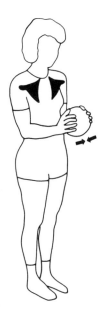

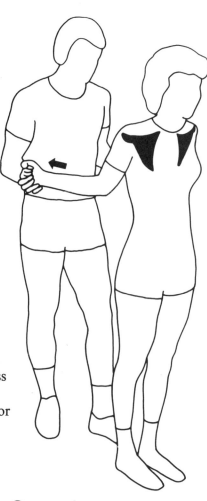

A. Tighten

Keep the elbow bent at 90 degrees with your upper arms close to the sides. Press your hands (with or without a ball) against each other as hard as possible for approximately 20 seconds.

B. Stretch

Move your arms backwards passively as far as possible with assistance of your practice partner. The upper arms are still kept close to your sides and the stretch is kept for 20 seconds.

Note: The exercise can also be done by yourself in a corner, a door frame or similar elsewhere.

7. The Forward Oscillators of the Arm —

M. coracobrachialis, m. deltoideus pars ventralis, m. pectoralis major, m. biceps caput breve.

Function: Move the arm in a pendulum move from the back forward.

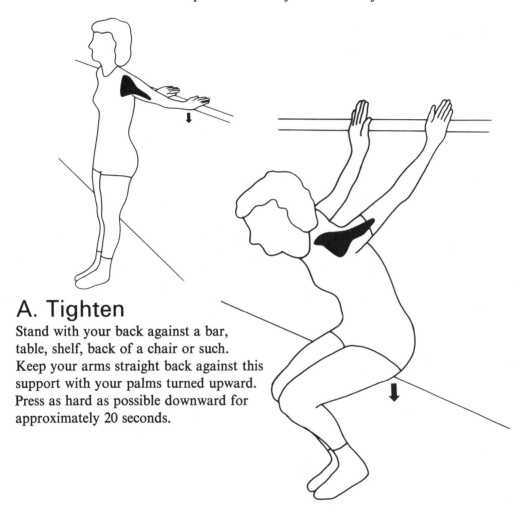

A. Tighten

Stand with your back against a bar, table, shelf, back of a chair or such. Keep your arms straight back against this support with your palms turned upward. Press as hard as possible downward for approximately 20 seconds.

B. Stretch

Keep your hands in the same position, but bend your knees and go down as far as possible. Feel the tightening in your shoulders, upper arms and chest. Keep the position for 15 seconds.

8. Muscles in the Back of the Shoulder ————————

M. deltoideus pars dorsalis, (m. latissimus dorsi, m. trapezius).

Function: *Move the arm backward when it is lifted in a 90-degree angle to the body and the elbow also bent 90 degrees.*

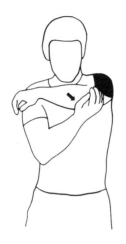

A. Tighten

Pull one elbow across the chest toward the other shoulder. From this position, press the elbow forward and out as hard as possible for 10–15 seconds using the other hand as resistance.

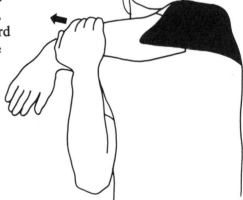

B. Stretch

Press your elbow as far as possible toward the other shoulder using your other assistant hand. Keep the stretch for 10–15 seconds.

9. Muscles in the Back of the Upperarm and Muscles in the Upper Side of the Back

M. triceps brachii caput longum, m. latissimus dorsi, m. deltoideus, m. teres major.

Function: Move the arm forward and downward from a raised elbow position.

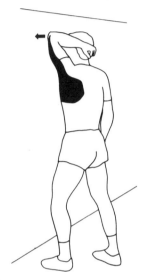

A. Tighten

Stand in front of a wall and raise the elbow, keeping the forearm straight back from the wall. Press the elbow as hard as possible against the wall for 15 seconds.

Alternative: You could also use the other hand as resistance, similar to the stretch picture.

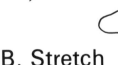

B. Stretch

Bend the arm backward and down toward the back using the other hand to press the elbow backward and downward. Keep the stretch for 15 seconds and feel the stretch in the back of the upper arm and upper part of your chest.

10. Muscles in the Back of the Upperarm and Muscles in the Back of the Shoulder —————

M. latissimus dorsi, m. deltoideus, m. triceps brachii.

Function: *Move the arm out and down from a raised position and extend the elbows.*

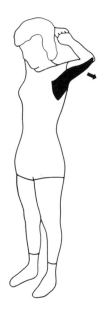

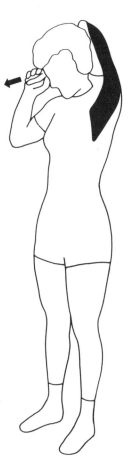

A. Tighten

Stand or sit with one elbow behind the neck. Try to pull your arm sideways and resist with the other hand. The easiest way to do this is to rest the helping hand or arm against your neck. Keep for approximately 20 seconds.

B. Stretch

Pull the arm (that was previously tightened in the opposite direction) behind your neck as far as possible using the helping hand. Keep in this position for 20 seconds.

Note: By bending further with the whole body, you can develop the exercise to a side-stretch (compare Exercise 52).

11. Forearm Muscles, "The Outside" (Extensors)

M. extensor digitorum, m. extensor digiti minimi, m. extensor carpi ulnaris, m. extensor carpi radialis longus & brevis, m. supinator.

Function: Bend upward (*extend*) in the wrist.

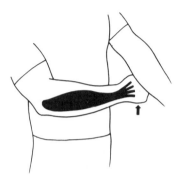

A. Tighten

Press your slightly tightened fist as hard as possible against the other arm or against the edge of a table, bar or such for approximately 20 seconds. Keep the elbow bent at a 90 degree angle.

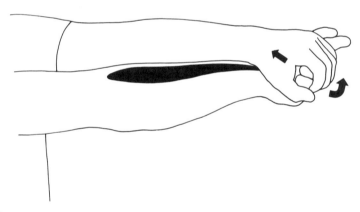

B. Stretch

Three steps: First bend the wrist downward as far as possible. Next extend the elbow and finally rotate the forearm inward as far as possible. At this point the fingers should be pointing out from the side ("Oriental waiter pose"). Then lift the arm in front of your body and hold on to the upper three fingers with the other hand and pull carefully up and back toward the body so that the tightening can be felt in the muscles on the "outside" or upper side of the forearm. Hold this position approximately 20 seconds.

12. Forearm Muscles, "The Inside" (Benders)

Mm. flexor digitorum superficialis & profundus, M. flexor pollicis longus, Mm. flexor carpi ulnaris & radialis.

Function: Bend (inward) in the wrist and the fingers.

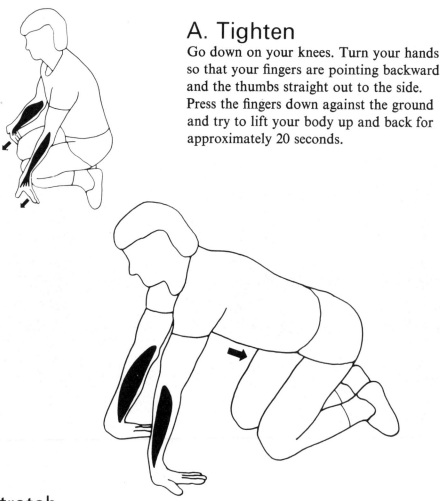

A. Tighten

Go down on your knees. Turn your hands so that your fingers are pointing backward and the thumbs straight out to the side. Press the fingers down against the ground and try to lift your body up and back for approximately 20 seconds.

B. Stretch

Stay in the kneeling position and place your hands with the fingers backward and thumbs to the side, a little distance in front of your knees. Move your body slightly backward so that you feel a tightening on the inside of your arm (now pointing forward). Keep the position for 20 seconds.

13. Forearm Muscles, "The Inside" (Benders)

Mm. flexor digitorum superficialis & profundus, m. flexor pollicis longus, Mm. flexor carpi ulnaris & radialis.

Function: Bend (inward) in the wrist and the fingers.

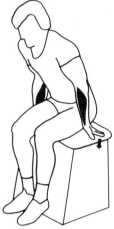

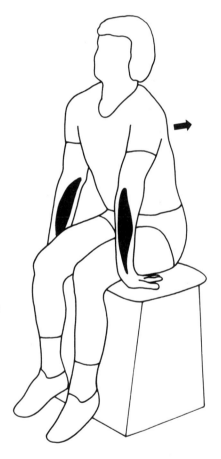

A. Tighten

Sit on a chair, vaulting horse or a bench, placing your hands on the seat, close to your sides fingers pointing backwards and with the thumbs straight out to the side. Press your fingers downward and forward as hard as possible and try to lift the body up and back for 20 seconds.

B. Stretch

Push the palms down onto the bench in the same position as before. Lean your upper body slowly backwards with your arms straight. Feel the tightening on the inside of the forearms. Keep for 20 seconds.

14. Forearm Muscles, "The Inside" (Benders)————

Mm. flexor digit. superfic. & profund., M. flexor pollicis longus, Mm. flexor carpi radialis & ulnaris, m. palmaris longus.

Function: Bend fingers and the wrist (inward).

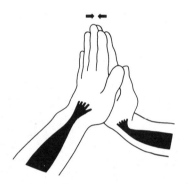

A. Tighten

Press your fingers against each other as hard as possible for 20 seconds. Let your palms be slightly apart.

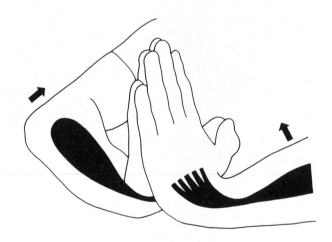

B. Stretch

Push the palms against each other and lift your elbows out and up with your arms in front of your chest. Feel the stretch on the inside of your forearm and keep it there for 20 seconds.

15. Forearm Muscles, "The Inside" (Benders)

Mm. flexor digit. superfic. & profund., Mm. flexor pollicis longus, Mm. flexor carpi radialis & ulnaris, m. palmaris longus.

Function: Bend fingers and the wrist.

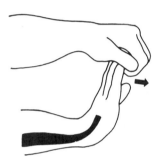

A. Tighten

Bend the wrist backwards and then press your fingers forward as far as possible using the other hand as resistance for 15 seconds.

B. Stretch

Bend your wrist backwards using the other hand to pull your fingers back and up. Keep in the furthest position for 15 seconds. Then switch and do the same exercise with the other hand.

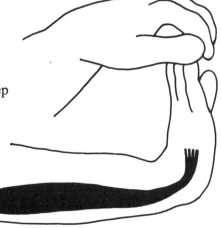

16.   Muscles in the Front of the Thigh—

M. quadriceps femoris.

Function: Bend (push outward and rotate inward) the hip and extend the knee.

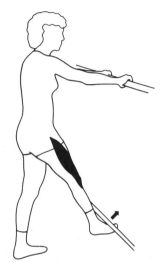

A. Tighten

Stand up with support for your hands.
Press one leg (with straight knee) forward
and upward as far as possible against
a bar, heavy piece of furniture or other
resistance for 20–30 seconds.

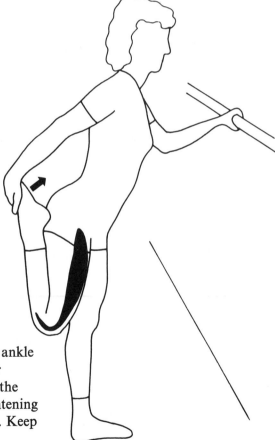

B. Stretch

Bend your knee and hold on to your ankle
with your hand. Move the foot as far
backward and up as possible so that the
heel reaches your buttocks and a tightening
is felt on the front side of your thigh. Keep
the stretch for 20–30 seconds.

17. The Muscles in the Front of the Thigh and the Hip

M. quadriceps femoris, m. iliopsoas.

Function: Bend the hip and extend the knee.

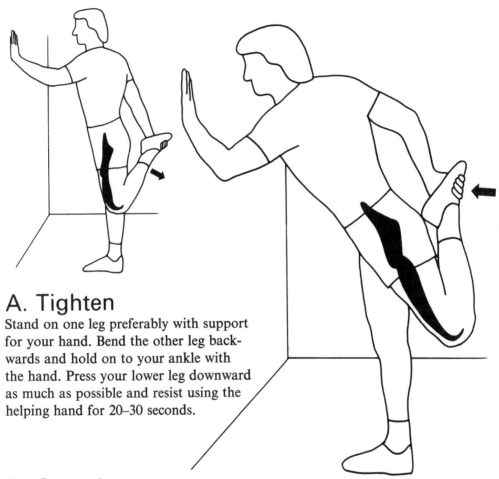

A. Tighten

Stand on one leg preferably with support for your hand. Bend the other leg backwards and hold on to your ankle with the hand. Press your lower leg downward as much as possible and resist using the helping hand for 20–30 seconds.

B. Stretch

Bend your knee and hold on to your ankle with your hand. Pull the foot as far backward and up as possible so that the heel reaches your buttocks and a tightening is felt on the front side of your thigh. Keep the stretch for 20–30 seconds.

Note: Consequently the stretch should preferably be made with the help of the hand on the opposite side grasping, far out on the foot, behind the back pulling your heel up toward your buttocks. By using the opposite hand for the stretch, the knee is bent in a more natural angle.

18. The Muscles in the Front of the Thigh and the Hip——————

M. quadriceps femoris, M. iliacus+m. psoas major=m. iliopsoas.

Function: Bend the hip and extend the knee.

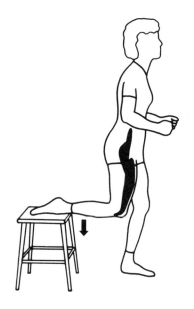

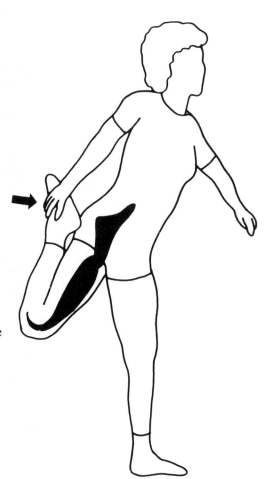

A. Tighten

Stand on one leg and with the other knee
bent, put the foot up behind you on a
chair or bar. Press your foot downward
as much as possible. Try to "push the
chair into the floor" for 20–30 seconds.
Keep supporting the other leg slightly
bent at the knee.

B. Stretch

Bend the knee and grab your ankle with one hand. Move the foot backward and
up as far as possible so that your heel touches the buttocks and you can feel a
tightening on the front of your thigh. Keep the stretch for 20–30 seconds.

19. The Muscles in the Front of the Thigh

M. quadriceps femoris.

Function: Bend the hip and extend the knee.

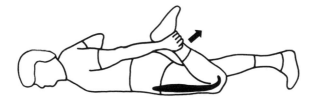

A. Tighten

Lie on your stomach and grab the ankle with the hand. Press the bent leg as hard as possible against the resisting hand for 20–30 seconds.

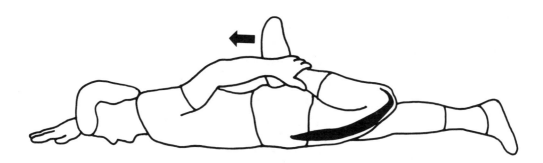

B. Stretch

Pull your lower leg upward and backward with your hand so that the heel touches your buttocks. Feel the tightening at the front of the thigh and keep it there for 20–30 seconds.

20. The Muscles in the Front of the Thigh and the Hip

M. quadriceps femoris, m. iliopsoas.

Function: Bend the hip and extend the knee.

Note: This exercise is done with a stretch position of the front of the lower leg and can therefore be combined with exercises for the muscles bending the foot joint upwards (see Exercises 43 and 44).

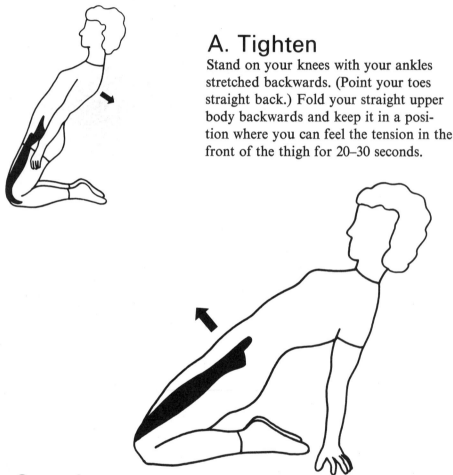

A. Tighten

Stand on your knees with your ankles stretched backwards. (Point your toes straight back.) Fold your straight upper body backwards and keep it in a position where you can feel the tension in the front of the thigh for 20–30 seconds.

B. Stretch

Fold your upper body further backwards and support yourself with your hands on the floor behind the body. Move your hips up as far as possible and feel the tightening on the front of the thigh and stay in that position 20–30 seconds.

21. The Muscles in the Back of the Thighs (Hamstrings)

M. biceps femoris, m. semitendinosus, m. semimembranosus (m. gracilis, m. sartorius).

Function: *Extend (and move inward) in the hip-joint and bend at the knee.*

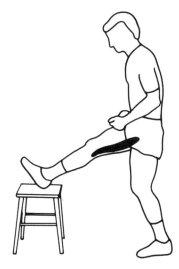

A. Tighten

Stand with one leg on a stool, or similar object, with your knee straight. Keep your body fairly straight but bend the other knee slightly. Press your heel against the stool as hard as possible and try to "push the chair through the floor" 20–30 seconds. Feel the tightening on the back side of the thigh.

B. Stretch

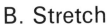

Bend forward at the hip keeping your back straight, which will be easier to do if you keep your head up and your hands on your back. The stretch is more effective if you bend the supporting leg more. Keep the position for 20–30 seconds.

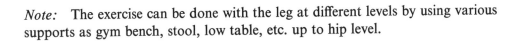

Note: The exercise can be done with the leg at different levels by using various supports as gym bench, stool, low table, etc. up to hip level.

22. The Muscles in the Back of the Thighs (Hamstrings)

M. biceps femoris, m. semitendinosus, m. semimembranosus.

Function: Extend (and move inward) the hip and bend the knee.

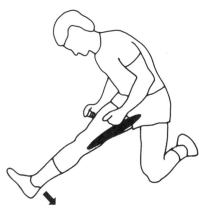

A. Tighten

Stand on one knee and keep the other leg almost straight out in front of you with your heel against the floor (hurdle sitting). Press the stretched out leg as hard as possible against the floor for 20–30 seconds and possibly support yourself with the other hand. Feel that the back of the thigh is tightened.

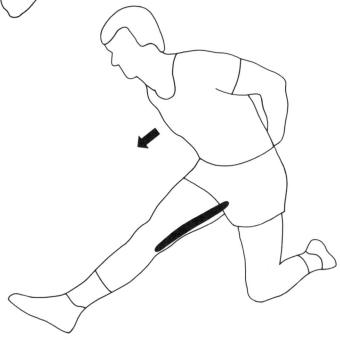

B. Stretch

Fold your upper body forward over the straight leg and keep your back as straight as possible. Keep your hands on your back if you like. Feel the stretch in the back of your thigh. Keep there for 20–30 seconds.

23. The Muscles in the Back of the Thighs (Hamstrings)——————

M. biceps femoris, m. semitendinosus, m. semimembranosus, m. gluteus maximus.

Function: Extend (and move inward) at the hip and bend at the knee.

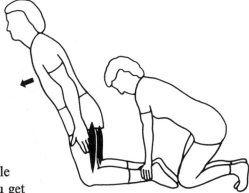

A. Tighten

Fold your upper body forward while standing on your knees, so that you get maximum tightening of the muscles in the back of your thighs and keep the position for 20–30 seconds. You will keep your balance by having your practice partner holding your feet to the ground or by pushing your feet under a heavy piece of furniture or similar object.

B. Stretch

Sit with your legs straight out in front of you and with your knees slightly bent. Stretch your arms forward and if you'd like grab your calves. Keep your back as straight as possible! Feel the stretch in the back of your thighs and keep there for 20–30 seconds.

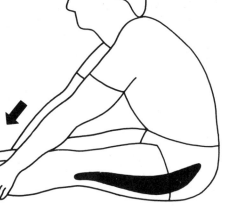

24. The Muscles in the Back of the Thighs (Hamstrings)

M. biceps femoris, m. semitendinosus, m. semimembranosus, m. gluteus maximus.

Function: Extend at the hip and bend at the knee.

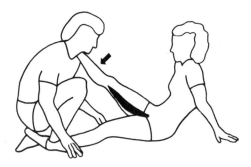

A. Tighten

Sit on the floor with your legs straight out in front and resting on your hands behind you. Put one leg on the shoulder of your practice partner and press down as much as possible for 20–30 seconds.

B. Stretch

Let your practice partner create a passive stretch by raising up slightly and therefore pushing your leg up. At the same time, your partner will push down on your knee to keep the knee straight. Feel the stretch on the back of the thigh and keep it there for 20–30 seconds.

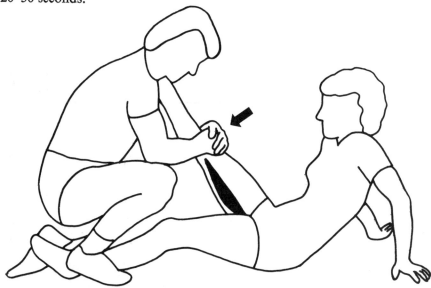

25. The Muscles in the Back of the Thighs (Hamstrings)—The Counteraction Method

M. biceps femoris caput longum, m. semitendinosus, m. semimembranosus, m. gluteus maximus, medius & minimus, m. tensor fasciae latae.

Function: *Extend the hip and rotate inward and move outward.*

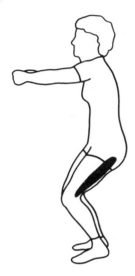

A. Tighten

Sit on the floor, preferably with support for your back, and bend and angle one of your legs up against your chest. Hold one hand around your ankle and the other around your knee. Stretch the other leg straight out. Press the knee and lower leg as hard as possible downwards with the two hands as resistance in 20 seconds.

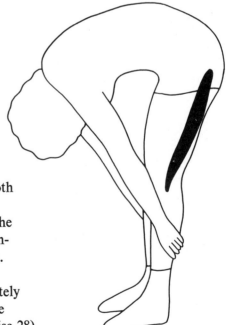

B. Stretch

Pull the leg up against your chest with both hands as far as you can and keep the position for 20 seconds. Make sure that the knee doesn't get any pressure. The tightening will be in the back of the upper thigh.

Note: If the stretch can't be felt adequately in the sitting position, this exercise can be done in a lying down position (see Exercise 28).

26. Muscles in the Back of the Thighs, Muscles in the Lower Back and Muscles in Your Buttocks —————

M. biceps femoris, m. semitendinosus, m. semimembranosus, M. gluteus maximus, m. adductor magnus.

Function: Extend at the hip.

A. Tighten

Lie down on your back with your lower back straight and your head on the floor. Bend one leg and clasp your hands around your knee. Press the knee downward as much as possible against the resisting hands for 20–30 seconds.

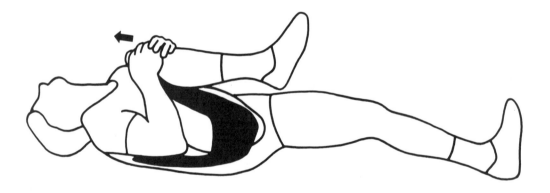

B. Stretch

Pull the bent leg up toward your head as far as possible with help from your clasped hands. Keep your lower back straight and keep your head on the floor. Keep the position for 20–30 seconds.

Variation: You can modify this exercise by turning the bent knee toward the opposite side of your chest.

27. The Muscles in the Front, Back and Outside of the Thigh and the Muscles in the Buttocks———

M. biceps femoris caput longum, m. semitendinosus, m. semimembranosus, m. gluteus maximus, medius & minimus, m. tensor fasciae latae.

Function: *Extend the hip and rotate inward and move outward.*

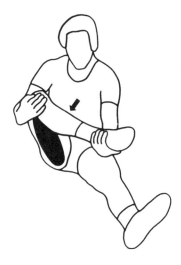

A. Tighten

Sit on the floor, preferably with support for your back, and bend and angle one of your legs up against your chest. Hold one hand around your ankle and the other around your knee. Stretch the other leg straight out. Press the knee and lower leg as hard as possible downwards with the two hands as resistance in 20 seconds.

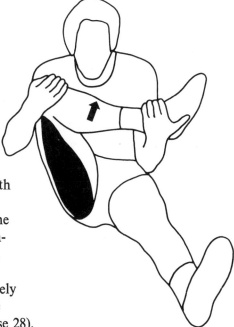

B. Stretch

Pull the leg up against your chest with both hands as far as you can and keep the position for 20 seconds. Make sure that the knee doesn't get any pressure. The tightening will be in the back of the upper thigh.

Note: If the stretch can't be felt adequately in the sitting position, this exercise can be done in a lying down position (see Exercise 28).

28. The Muscles in the Front, Back and Outside of the Thigh and the Muscles in the Buttocks ————————

M. biceps femoris, m. semitendinosus, m. semimembranosus, m. gluteus maximus, medius & minimus, m. tensor fasciae latae.

Function: *Extend the hip and rotate inward and move outward.*

A. Tighten

Lie down on your back and bring your bent leg up against your chest. Grab your ankle with one hand and the knee with the other. Press your leg down and out with your hands providing resistance for 20 seconds. Keep the other leg straight out.

Note: There should be no strain or pressure on the knee. The tightening should be felt in the back of the upper thigh.

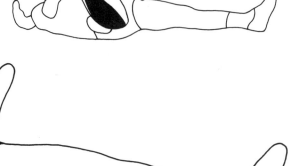

B. Stretch

Pull the leg up against your chest as far as you can and keep it there for 20 seconds with the leg more or less crosswise over your chest. The other leg should be straight out on the floor.

29. Outside Hip Muscles————————

M. tensor fasciae latae, m. gluteus medius & minimus, m. gemellus sup. & inf., m. piriformis, m. quadratus femoris, m. obturatorius int. & ext.

Function: Push outward at the hip.

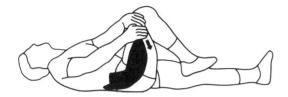

A. Tighten

Lie down on your back and bend your leg to a 90-degree angle. Press your thigh out to the side as much as you can for 20 seconds using both hands or a wall as resistance. Keep your feet and ankles relaxed.

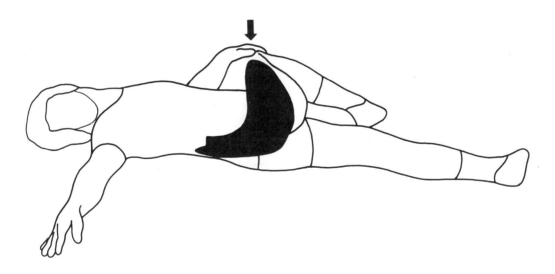

B. Stretch

Pull your leg up over the other one and down toward the floor using the opposite hand. Keep the position for 20 seconds with your shoulders still touching the floor. Rest the other hand straight out to the side and turn your head the same way so that you can watch that hand.

30. Outside Hip Muscles and Muscles in the Buttocks————————

M. tensor fasciae latae, m. sartorius, m. piriformis, m. gemellus sup. & inf., m. obturatorius int., m. gluteus medius & minimus.

Function: Move the hip outward and rotate the hip outward. "Secretary stretch" This exercise should be done after the groin stretch (see Exercises 31–35).

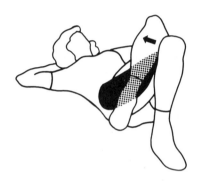

A. Tighten

Lie down on your back with your hands behind your neck. Bend your knees and lift one leg up over the other. The bottom leg should be turned somewhat down and in. Then press the lower leg up and out as far as possible for 20 seconds using the crossed-over leg as resistance.

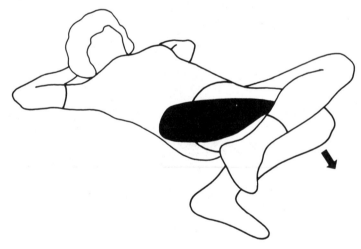

B. Stretch

Stretch the bottom leg down toward the floor and let the weight of the upper leg press down on the lower one. The tightening should be felt on the outer side of your hip. Keep the position for 20–30 seconds.

31. The Groin Muscles, "The Inside" of the Thigh (The Adductors)———

M. adductor longus & brevis, m. adductor magnus, m. gracilis, m. pectineus.

Function: Move in the hip inward (bend and rotate outward). "Tailor Stretch"

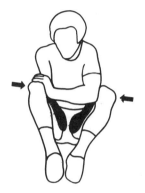

A. Tighten

Sit on the floor with knees bent and move your feet back toward your buttocks. Keep your knees apart by holding your ankles or placing a ball between your knees or (as in the picture) placing your forearms straight across. Press your knees against each other as hard as possible for 20–30 seconds.

B. Stretch

Move your heels toward your buttocks by pulling your ankles closer. Push lightly with your elbows to move your knees out to the side as far as possible. Bend your upper body slightly forward and keep the stretch (which will be felt along the insides of the thighs) for 20–30 seconds.

32. The Groin Muscles, "The Inside" of the Thigh (The Adductors)

M. adductor longus & brevis, m. adductor magnus, m. gracilis, m. pectineus.

Function: *Move in the hip inward (bend and rotate outward).*

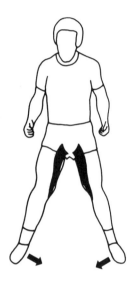

A. Tighten

Stand with your feet wide apart and if available, support yourself from a bar, table or chair. Tighten the inside of your thighs by pressing the insides of your feet down and in as hard as possible toward the floor for 20–30 seconds.

B. Stretch

Slide your feet out sideways and stop in the furthest position you can for 20–30 seconds.

Note: From this outside position, another identical move can be made to get yet a little further out as well as in Exercise 31.

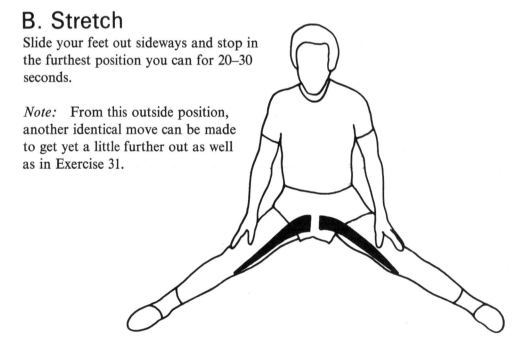

33. The Groin Muscles, "The Inside" of the Thigh (The Adductors)———

M. adductor longus & brevis, m. adductor magnus, m. gracilis, m. pectineus.

Function: *Move in the hip inward (bend and rotate outward).*

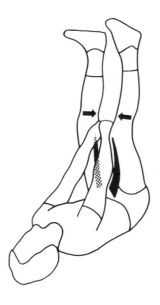

A. Tighten

Lie down on your back with your legs straight up against the wall. Press your legs together as hard as possible with (for example) your hands between your knees for 20–30 seconds.

Tip: The starting position is easily reached by placing your buttocks 4–6 inches from the wall and both legs to one side. Then lift the legs into position. Use a surface where you won't slip.

B. Stretch

Spread your legs slowly as far as possible. "Hang" passively with straight legs and your heels against the wall for 20–30 seconds. The support from the wall makes it possible to keep the stretch longer in a stable relaxed position.

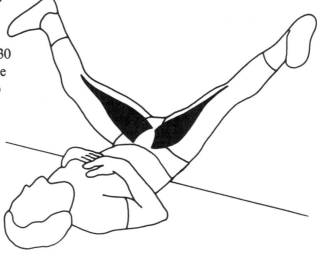

34. The Groin Muscles, "The Inside" of the Thigh (The Adductors)———

M. adductor longus & brevis, m. adductor magnus, m. gracilis, m. pectineus.

Function: *Move in the hip inward (bend and rotate outward).*

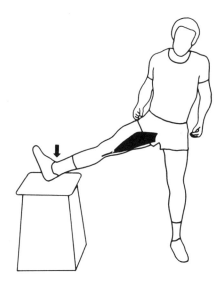

A. Tighten

Stand on one leg with the other leg stretched out sideways and with the heel resting on a gym horse, tall chair or similar object. Press your heel down as hard as possible and try to "pushing the support into the floor" for 20–30 seconds. Keep your upper body and the supporting foot facing forward. Feel free to support yourself with the opposite hand on a chair back, wall, etc.

Tip: Stretch the tightest, least flexible side first.

B. Stretch

Bend slowly straight sideways toward the stretched out leg and keep the position for 20–30 seconds. In order to accentuate the stretch, you can bend the supporting leg a little at the knee.

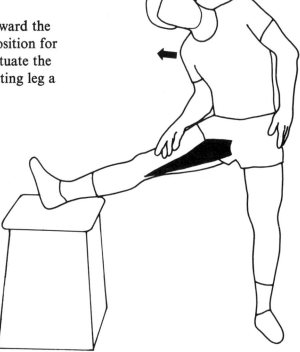

35. The Groin Muscles, "The Inside" of the Thigh (The Adductors)———

M. adductor longus & brevis, m. adductor magnus, m. gracilis, m. pectineus.

Function: Move in the hip inward (bend and rotate outward).

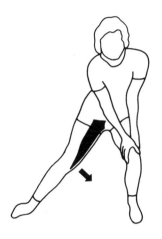

A. Tighten

Stand with one leg almost bent to a 90-degree angle and the other leg straight out to the side. Press the straightened leg toward the floor as hard as possible and feel the inside of your thigh tighten for 20–30 seconds. Use the bent knee as a rest for your hands.

Alternative: This part of the exercise can also be done standing on your knees supported by your hands against a wall, a chair, etc.

B. Stretch

Slide out sideways with the straight leg and/or bend the supporting leg further. Keep your back as straight as possible. Feel the tightening on the inside of the thigh. Keep the position for 20–30 seconds.

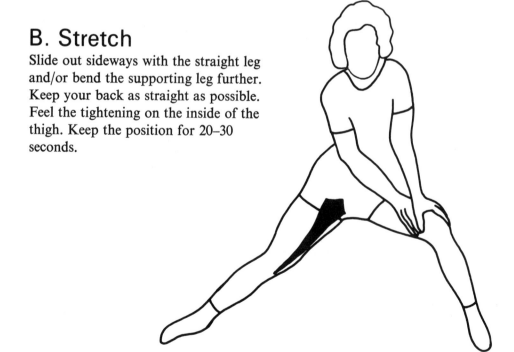

36. The Deep Hip Bending Muscles——

M. psoas major, m. iliacus (m. sartorius, m. quadriceps, adductors).

Function: Bend at the hip.

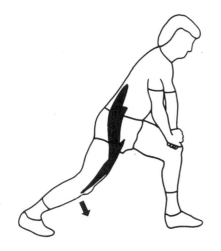

A. Tighten

Stand with one foot relatively far behind you ("long-walk-standing") and rest your hands on the other knee, bar, chair, etc. Press the back leg "through the floor" as hard as possible for 20–30 seconds.

B. Stretch

Move your hip forward, keeping the upper body straight up and the back leg stretched out. Feel the tightening in the hip and keep the position for 20–30 seconds. The stretch can be accentuated by putting the back knee on the ground.

Note: Don't keep the front knee at such an angle that it is in front of the ankle, since this hinders the real stretch in the hip.

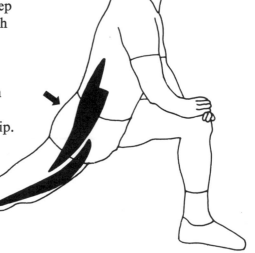

Alternative: This exercise can also be done with the back leg on a gym bench, low chair or a stool. Normally, you will need support for your hand.

37. The Muscles Bending the Hips————

M. iliopsoas, m. quadriceps.

Function: Bend at the hip and extend at the knee.

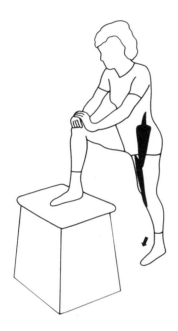

A. Tighten
Stand with one foot on a gym horse or a chair resting your hands on the knee of the same leg. Press the foot of the other leg forward and downward "through the floor" for 20–30 seconds.

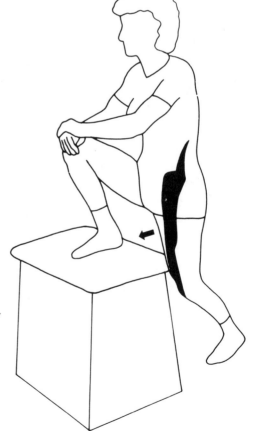

B. Stretch
Push your hip forward as far as possible keeping your feet in the same position. Feel the tightening in the groin/hip. Stay in that position 20–30 seconds.

38. The Calf Muscles

M. gastrocnemius+m. soleus=m. triceps surae, m. fibularis longus & brevis, m. tibialis posterior, m. flexor digitorum longus, m. flexor hallucis longus.

Function: *Bend (downward) at the ankle, middle foot joints and the toe joints or, in other words, all the bending mechanisms of the foot and the ankle.*

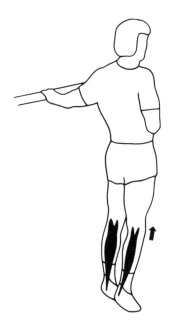

A. Tighten

Tighten your calf muscles by standing up on your toes as high as possible. Feel the tightening in the calf and keep it there 20–30 seconds. Get strong hand support at waist height from a bar or a similar object.

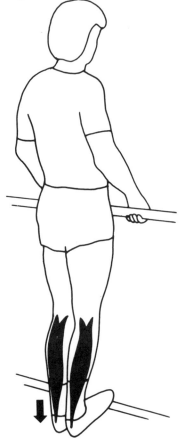

B. Stretch

Stand with the front part of the foot bottoms on a bar or a high edge and let the heels sink downward as far as possible. Feel the stretch in the calf and keep the position for 20–30 seconds. Take a firm hand support on a bar or something corresponding in waist level.

39. The Calf Muscles

M. gastrocnemius+m. soleus, m. fibularis longus & brevis, m. tibialis posterior, m. flexor digitorum longus, m. hallucis longus.

Function: Bend (downward) all the joints of the foot and the ankle.

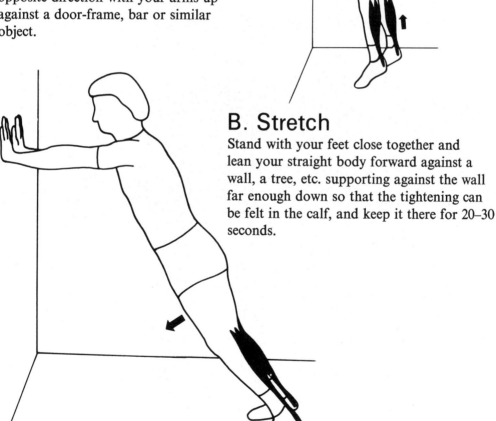

A. Tighten

Stand as high as possible on the tip of your toes for 20–30 seconds, preferably with hand support for better balance. To get maximum results, push in the opposite direction with your arms up against a door-frame, bar or similar object.

B. Stretch

Stand with your feet close together and lean your straight body forward against a wall, a tree, etc. supporting against the wall far enough down so that the tightening can be felt in the calf, and keep it there for 20–30 seconds.

40. The Calf Muscles ───────────────

M. gastrocnemius, m. soleus, m. tibialis posterior (o. m. plantaris).

Function: Bend (downward) the ankle.

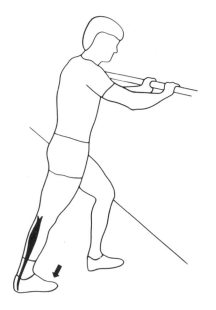

A. Tighten

Lean against a bar, a wall, a pole or a
tree with your hands at chest height and
your back foot approximately 2 feet
away from the object. Lean your body
slightly forward and stretch the back
leg until a slight tightening is felt.
Press the front of your foot or toes
against the ground as hard as possible
for 20–30 seconds. You could also raise
on the toes on the back foot while lifting
the front foot from the ground.

B. Stretch

Lean your body forward and move the hip
forward, making the back leg stretch
further. Feel the stretch in the calf and
keep it for 20–30 seconds.

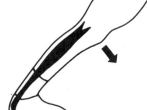

41. The Calf Muscles and the Achilles Tendon with Bent Knee ────────

M. soleus, m. fibularis longus & brevis, m. flexor digit. longus, m. flexor hallucis longus, m. tibialis posterior.

Function: Bend (downward) in the foot and the ankle.

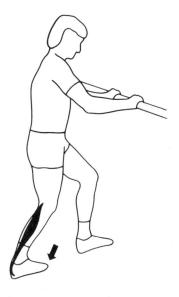

A. Tighten

Lean in a "walk-standing" position against a wall, bar or tree with the back leg bent and the foot approximately 2 feet away from the object. Press your toes against the ground as hard as possible for 20–30 seconds.

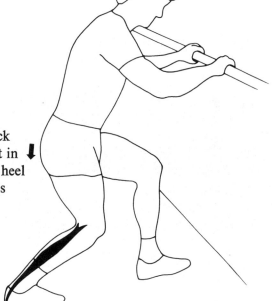

B. Stretch

Sink down at the hip and move the back knee forward so that a tightening is felt in the lower portion of the calf. Keep the heel on the ground during the 20–30 seconds stretch.

Alternative: The "Achilles stretch" can also be done in kneeling position with one leg at a time and the other ankle extended against the floor in "toe-pointing backward." Bend the actual leg forward and put the foot bottom against the floor and let the heel leave the floor 4–9 inches. Then move the thigh forward in a smooth movement so that you feel the stretch in the Achilles tendon. Keep the position for at least 15 seconds with your hands support on the floor in front of the rest of the body.

42. The Calf Muscles—The Counter-action Method ———————

M. triceps surae, m. tibialis posterior, m. fibularis longus & brevis, m. flexor digit. longus, m. flexor hallucis longus.

Function: Bend (downward) in the ankle, middle foot joint and the toe joints.

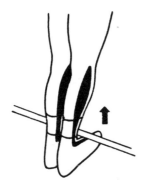
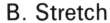

A. Tighten

Tighten the upward extensor muscles of the feet (that counteract the calf muscles) as hard as possible with resistance, for example, by standing on the heels and raising the toes up as far as you can preferably with a heavy piece of furniture as resistance.

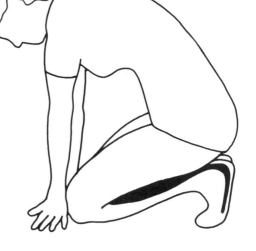

B. Stretch

Stretch passively by sitting down on your knees with the toes touching the ground for 20–30 seconds.

43. The Muscles in the Front of the Lower Leg————————

M. tibialis anterior, m. extensor digitorum longus, m. extensor hallucis longus.

Function: Bend upward (extend) in the ankle and the toe joints.

A. Tighten

Tighten the upward extensor muscles
of the feet (that counteract the calf
muscles) as hard as possible with
resistance, for example, by standing on
the heels and raising the toes up as
far as you can preferably with a heavy
piece of furniture as resistance.

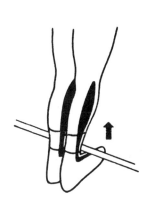
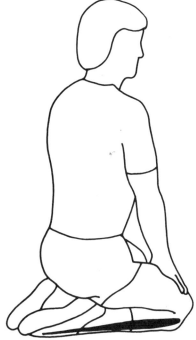

B. Stretch

Sit down on your knees with your heels under your buttocks, and your toes
pointing straight back. Keep the position for 20–30 seconds. The exercise can be
accentuated by leaning your body backwards.

Tip: This exercise could preferably be combined with Exercise 20 for the
muscles bending the hip and the muscles in the front of the thighs.

44. The Toes Upward Benders (Extensors)

M. extensor digit. longus, m. extensor hallucis longus, m. extensor digit. brevis, m. extensor hallucis brevis, m. tibialis anterior.

Function: Bend upward (extend) in the toe joints.

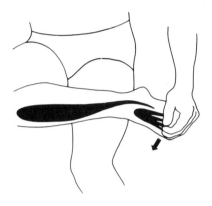

A. Tighten

Sit with one leg angled over the thigh of the other leg and your foot moved somewhat inward (supinated). Grab the top side of the toes and press them upward as hard as possible for 20–30 seconds using your hand as resistance.

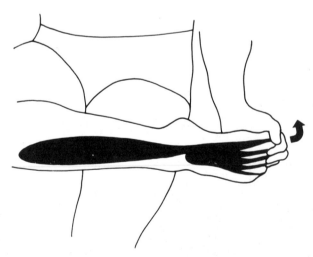

B. Stretch

Pull with your hand so that your toes bend downward as far as possible. The ankle will stretch also. Keep in this position for 20–30 seconds.

45. The Toes Downward Benders (Flexors)

M. flexor digit. longus & brevis, m. flexor hallucis longus & brevis, mm. lumbricales.

Function: Bend (downward) in the middle foot joints, the basic toe joints (MTP) and the toe joints (PIP, DIP)

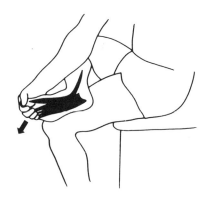

A. Tighten

Sit with one leg angled over the thigh of the other leg. Press your toes actively downward as hard as possible using the hand on the same side as resistance. The ankle is angled upward. Keep in this position for 20–30 seconds.

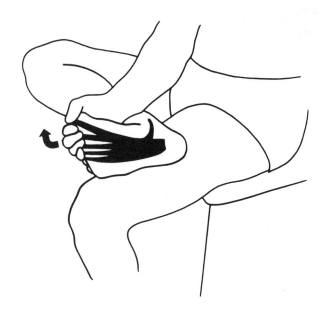

B. Stretch

Move your toes passively upward as far as possible by pulling all the toes upward with your hand. The ankle will then also be angled upward. Hold for 20–30 seconds.

46. The Deep Back Muscles—The Extensors

Mm. erectores spinae=m. iliocostalis cervicis, thoracis & lumborum+m. longissimus cervicis, thoracis & capitis+m. semispinalis capitis, Mm. interspinales, m. spinalis.

Function: Extend the back, bend the spinal column backwards.

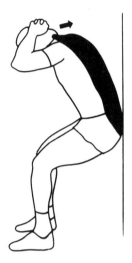

A. Tighten

Stand up leaning slightly forward so that your back doesn't sway. Lean with your lower back against a wall with your knees slightly bent. Clasp your hands behind your neck and press your back backwards as hard as possible using your hands and for example the wall behind as resistance for 20–30 seconds.

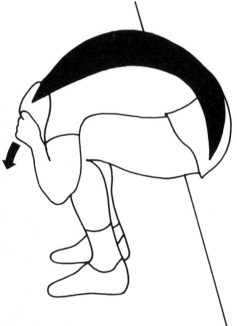

B. Stretch

Bend your back forward (with some help from your hands) and feel the tightening along the spine. Keep in this position for 20–30 seconds.

Alternative: This exercise can also be done sitting down with knees bent and your head between your knees.

47. The Back Extensors Muscles————

Mm. erectores truncii, m. trapezius.

Function: Extending the back and bend the spinal column backwards.

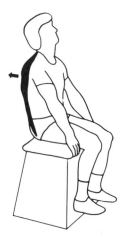

A. Tighten

"Static rowing": Sit down and grab the seat of the chair, the gym horse top, etc. Fold your body backwards and try as hard as possible to move the seat back under your body for 20–30 seconds.

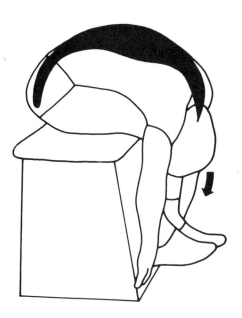

B. Stretch

Fold your upper body forward and downward, and hang passively in this position for 20–30 seconds.

48. The Deep Back Muscles, The Extensor Layer

Mm. erectores spinae.

Function: Extend the back, bend the spinal column backwards.

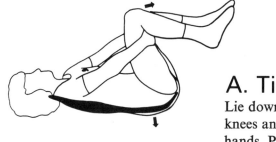

A. Tighten

Lie down on your back, pull up your knees and grab under them with your hands. Push your buttocks against the floor and press your knees downward as hard as possible, using your hands as resistance, for approximately 20 seconds.

B. Stretch

Pull your knees up as far as possible against your chin and keep the position for 20 seconds.

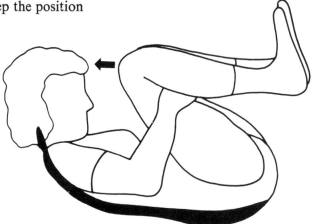

70

49. The Neck Muscles

Mm. iliocostalis cervicis, m. longissimus capitis & cervicis, m. semispinalis capitis, cervicis & thoracis och Mm. nuchae profundii=mm. rectus capitis posterior minor & major+mm. obliquus capitis superior & inferior, mm. interspinalis, m. multifidus cervicis, m. splenius capitis & cervicis.

Function: Bend the head backwards.

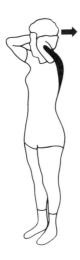

A. Tighten

Clasp your hands behind your neck and press as hard as possible against your hands as resistance for 20 seconds.

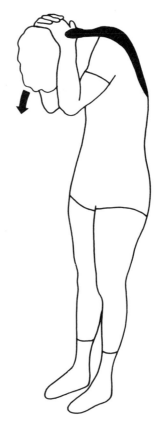

B. Stretch

Bend your head forward and pull down carefully with the help of your hands so that your chin touches the chest. Feel the stretch in your neck and keep in this position for approximately 20 seconds.

50. The Muscles of the Upper Back and the Neck———————

Mm. erectores spinae, Mm. nuchae profundii, M. splenius capitis & cervicis, M. transversospinalis.

Function: Bend the head and the neck backwards.

A. Tighten

Lie down on your back with your knees pulled up and your hands clasped behind your neck. Lift your head up slightly and then press backwards actively as hard as you can against your clasped hands for approximately 20 seconds.

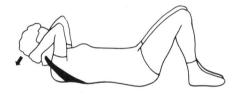

B. Stretch

Pull your head up and forward using your clasped hands, so that the tightening is felt in the neck muscles and in your upper back. Keep in this position for approximately 20 seconds.

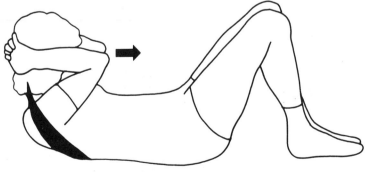

51. The Muscles on the Side of the Neck

M. scalenus anterior, medius & posterior, M. splenius capitis & cervicis, M. rectus capitis lateralis, M. spinalis capitis & cervicis, M. semispinalis capitis & cervicis, Mm. intertransversarii.

Function: Bend the neck sideways.

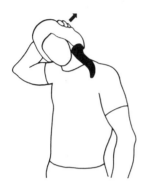

A. Tighten

Bend your head a little sideways and then press it back toward the other side. Resist by using the hand on the same side to hold your head. Maintain the tension for approximately 20 seconds.

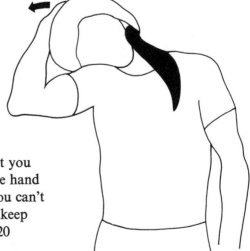

B. Stretch

Pull your head to the same side that you did the slight side bend to, using the hand or your head. Pull carefully until you can't go any further, feel the stretch and keep in that position for approximately 20 seconds.

52. The Muscles on the Side of Your Body ──────────

M. spinalis thoracis, M. obliquus externus & internus abdominis, M. quadratus lumborum, (m. triceps brachii).

Function: Bend the upper and lower part of the spinal column sideways.

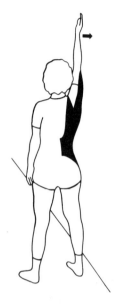

A. Tighten

Stand with your side against a wall. Keep your feet shoulder-width apart. Lift the arm next to the wall as high up as possible and press your handback and arm against the wall for 10–15 seconds.

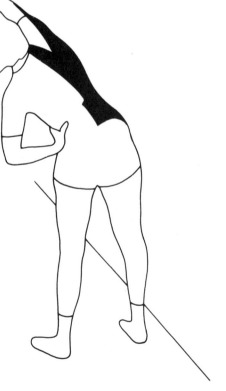

B. Stretch

Bend slowly at the waist away from the wall, keeping your arm straight over your head. Place the other hand on your hip and keep the stretch when you can feel it in your side. Hold for 10–15 seconds. Breathe out when going into the stretch.

Note: Go out of the stretch slowly, no jerky moves!

53. The Stomach Muscles————————

M. rectus abdominis huvudsakligen, dessutom, m. obliquus externus & internus abdominis, m. psoas major & minor.

Function: Bend (forward) in the chest and the lower back.

A. Tighten

Tighten your stomach muscles by raising up from a lying down position, and stop at a 30-degree angle to the floor in a "frozen sit-up" for 20–30 seconds. Preferably keep your hands on your thighs and knees slightly bent.

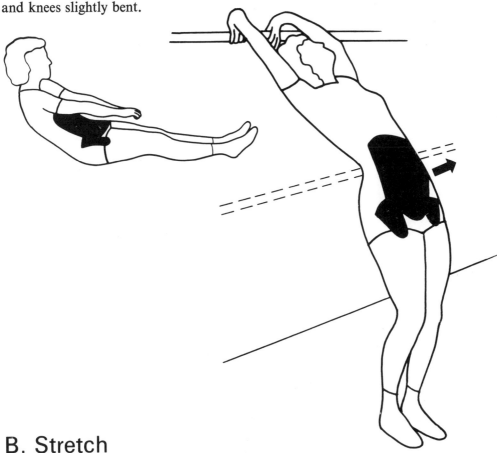

B. Stretch

Bend your trunk backwards, preferably over a support for your back (bar, table etc.) roughly 4–5 inches higher than your belly-button level. If no such support is available, get support from your hands by holding on to a wall behind you. Keep the stretch for 20–30 seconds.

Basic Program for Different Types of Sports ——

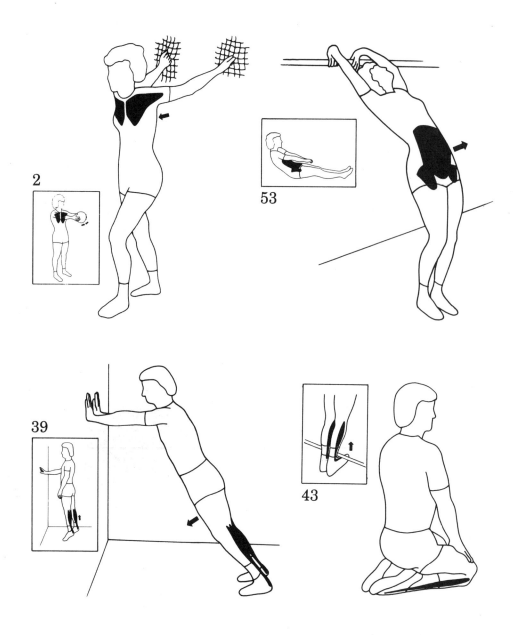

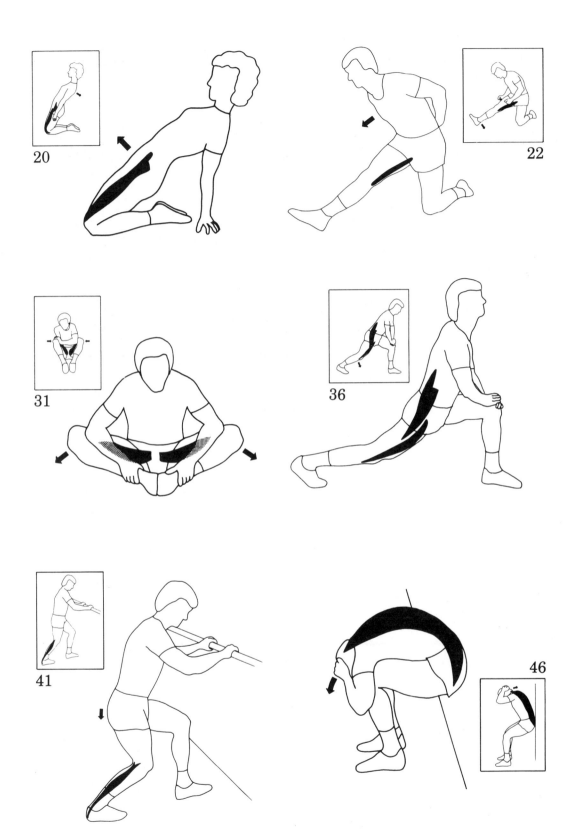

20

22

31

36

41

46

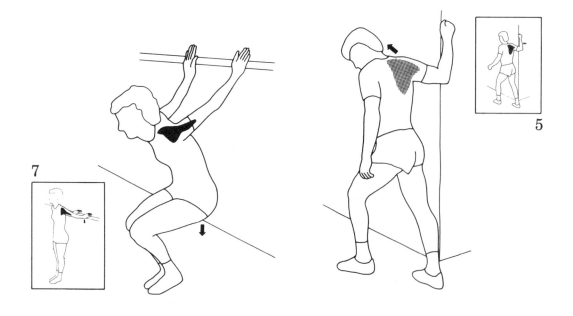

7

5

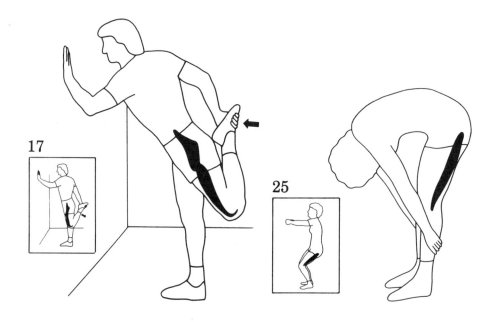

17

25

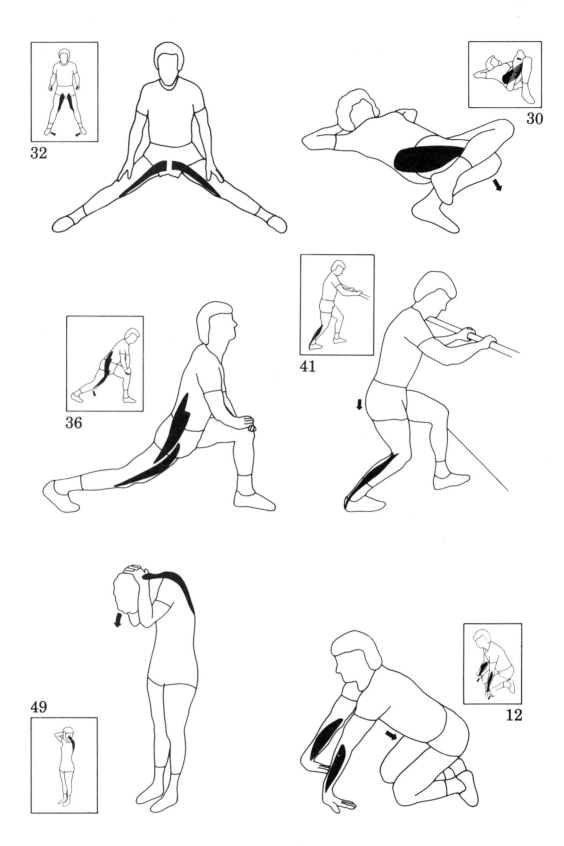

32

30

36

41

49

12

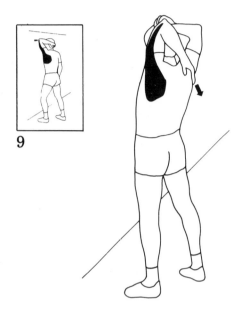

9

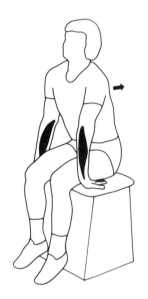

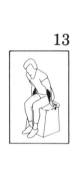

13

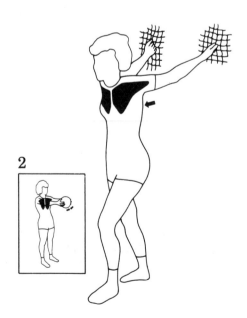

2

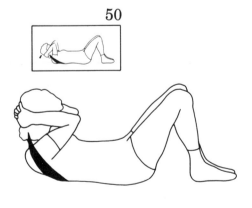

50

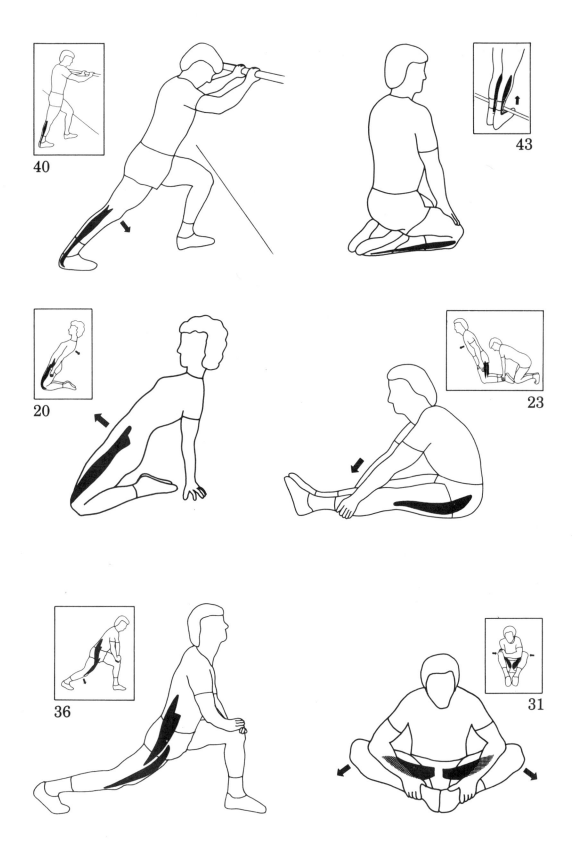

40

43

20

23

36

31

83

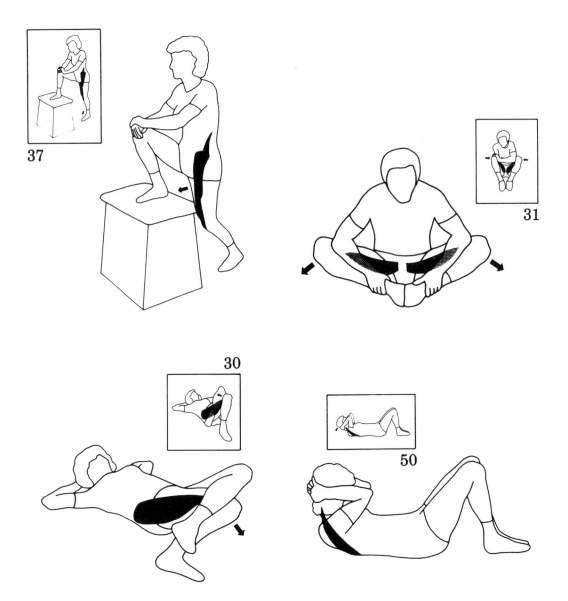

37

31

30

50

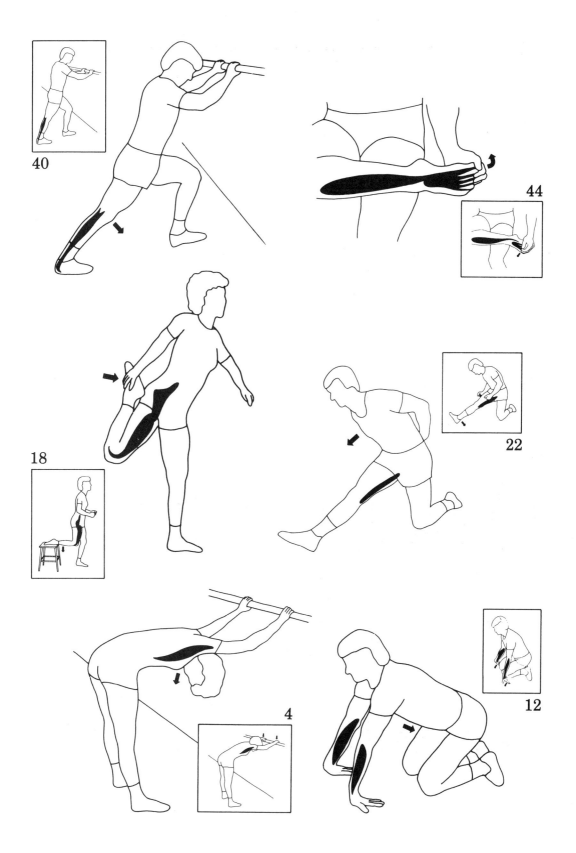

40

44

18

22

4

12

85

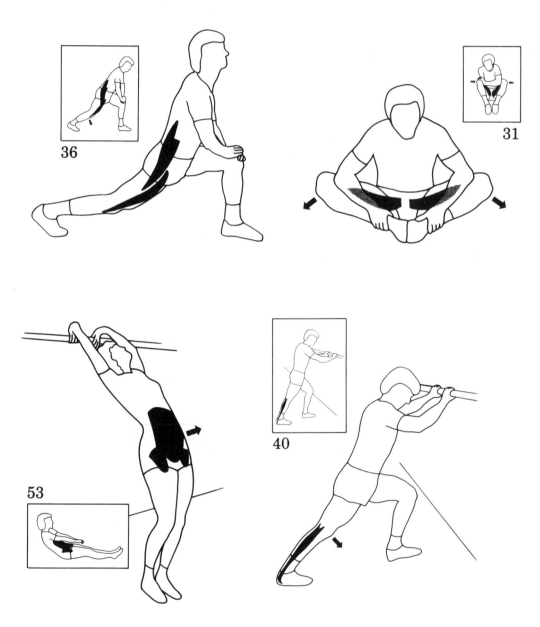

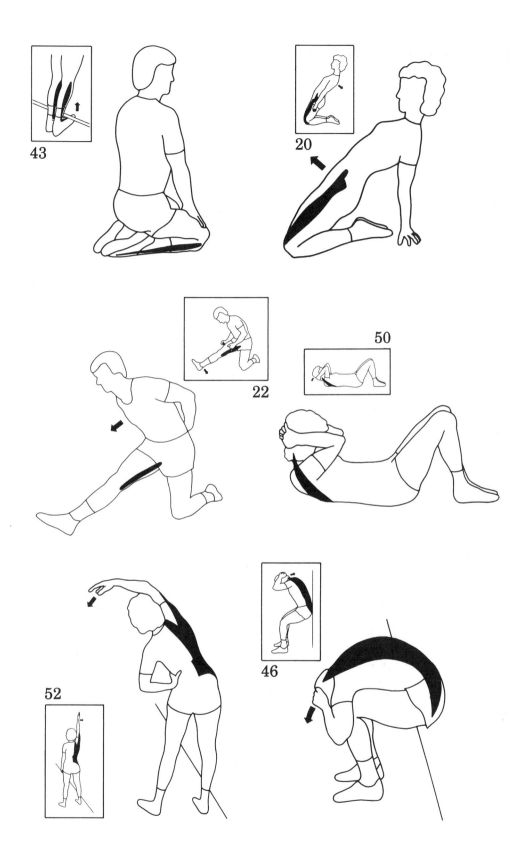

43

20

22

50

52

46

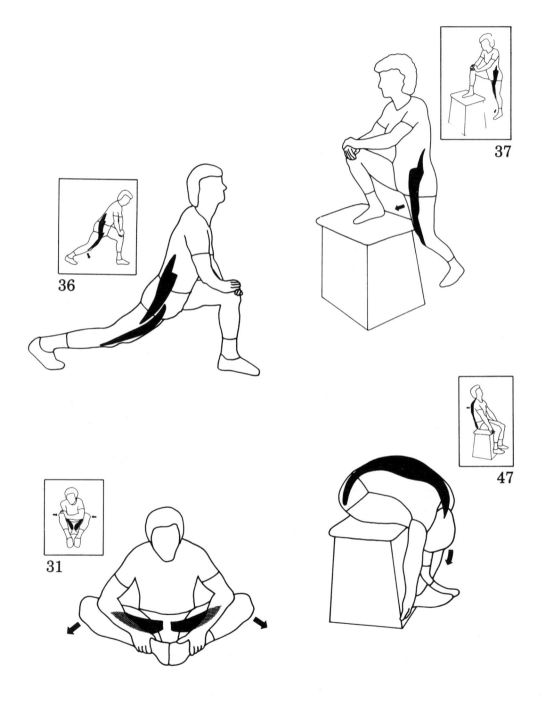

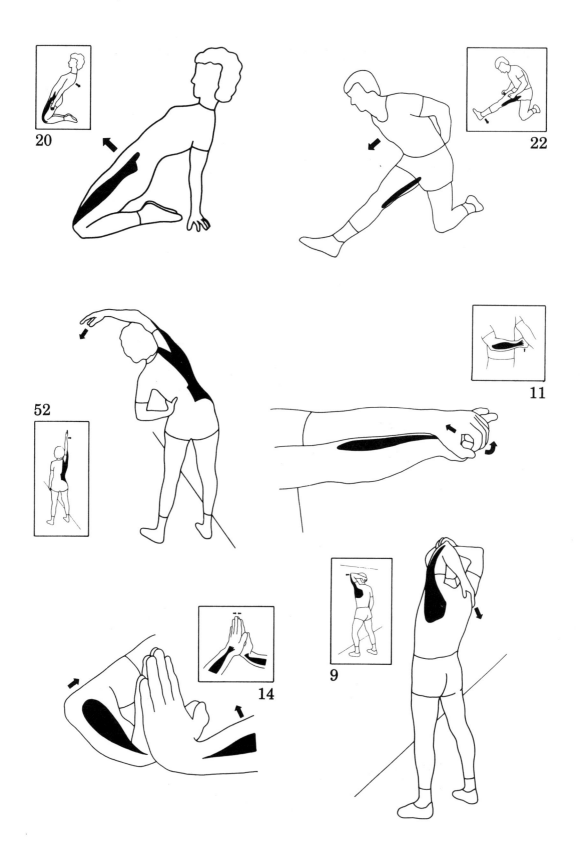

20

22

52

11

14

9

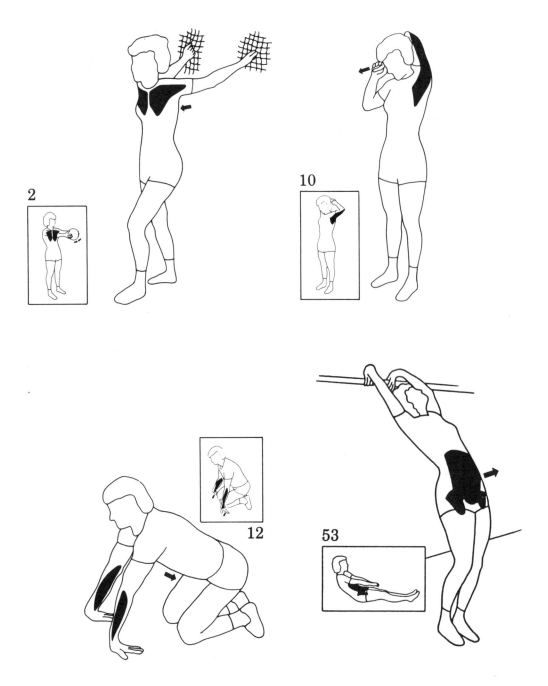

2

10

12

53

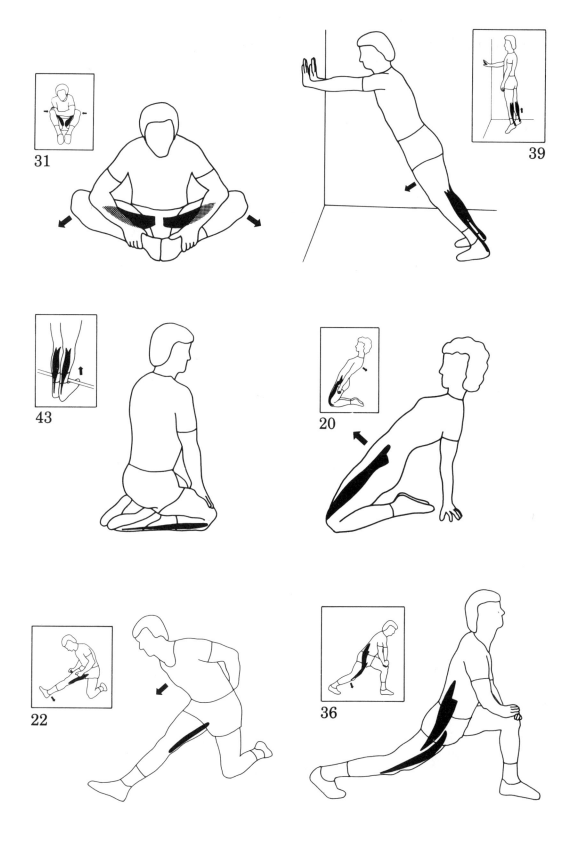

31

39

43

20

22

36

91

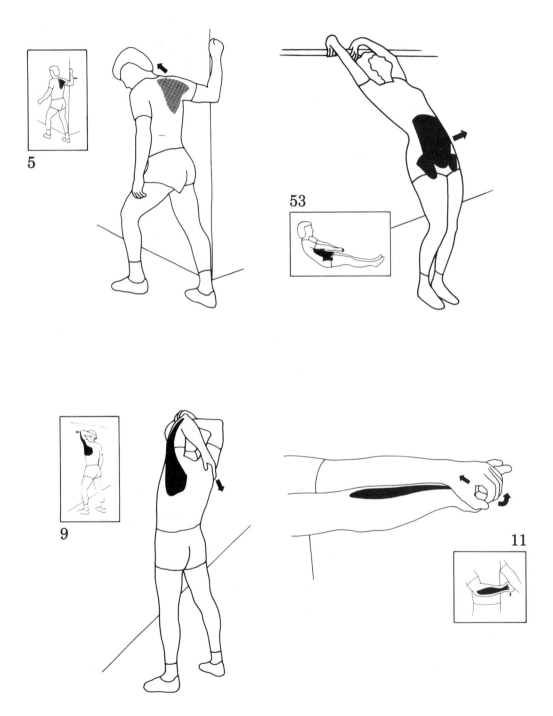

5

53

9

11

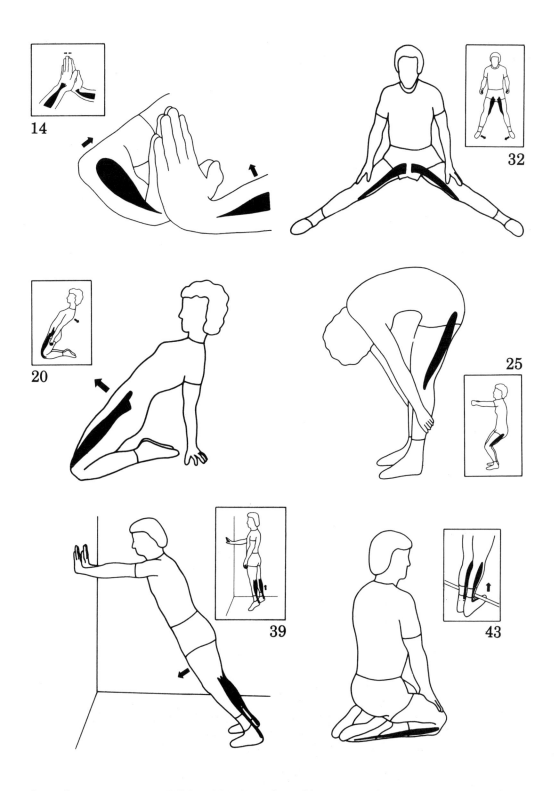

Special tennis exercise: With racket in point-of-impact position: Muscle tightening-stretch.

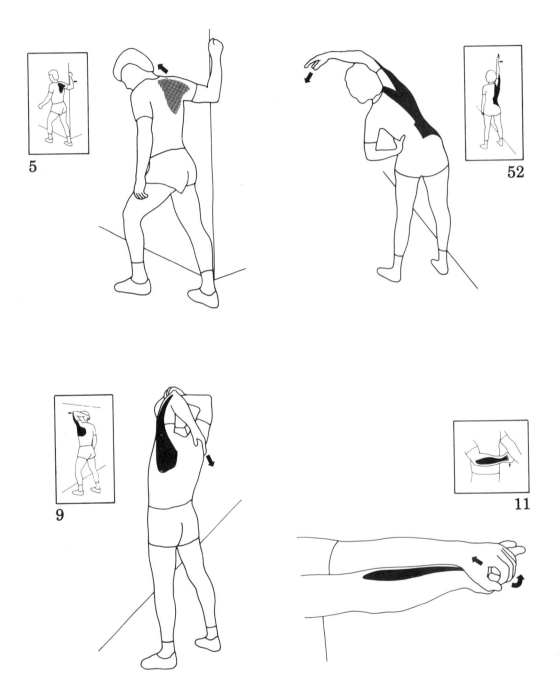

5

52

9

11

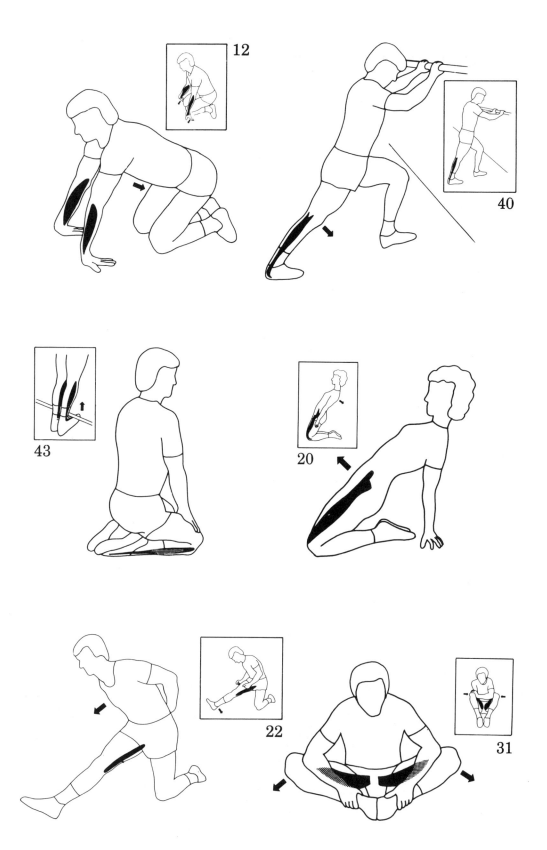

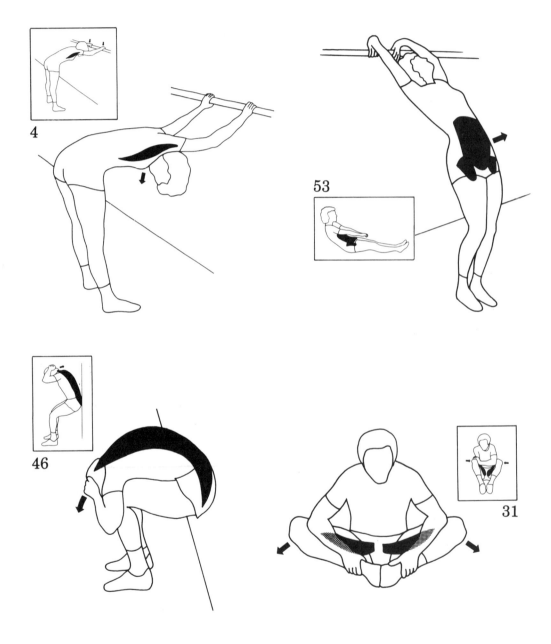

4

53

46

31

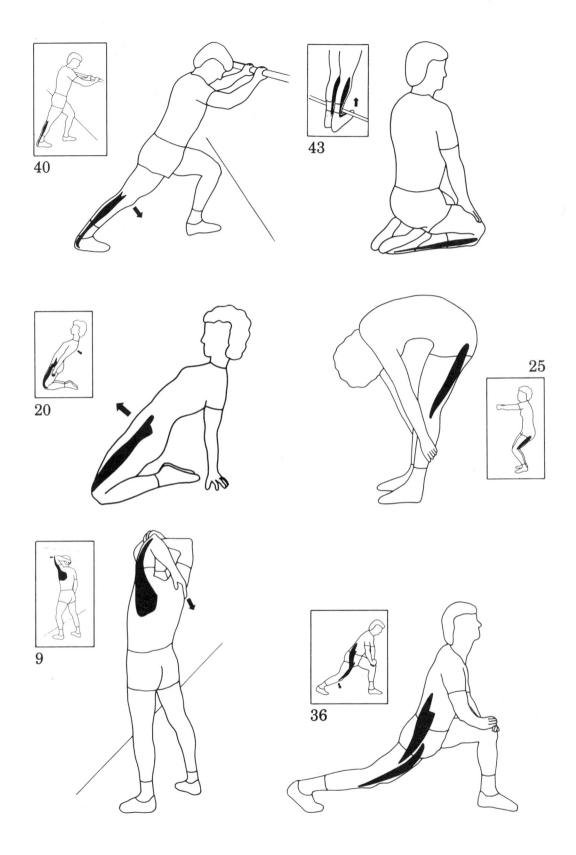

40

43

20

25

9

36

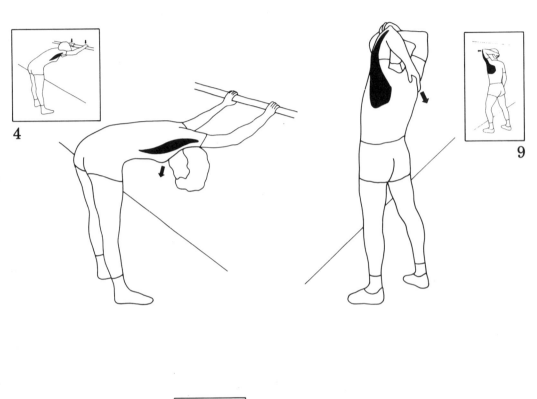

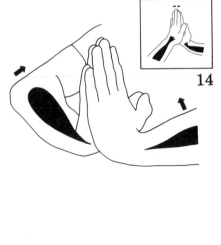

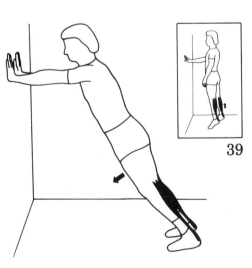

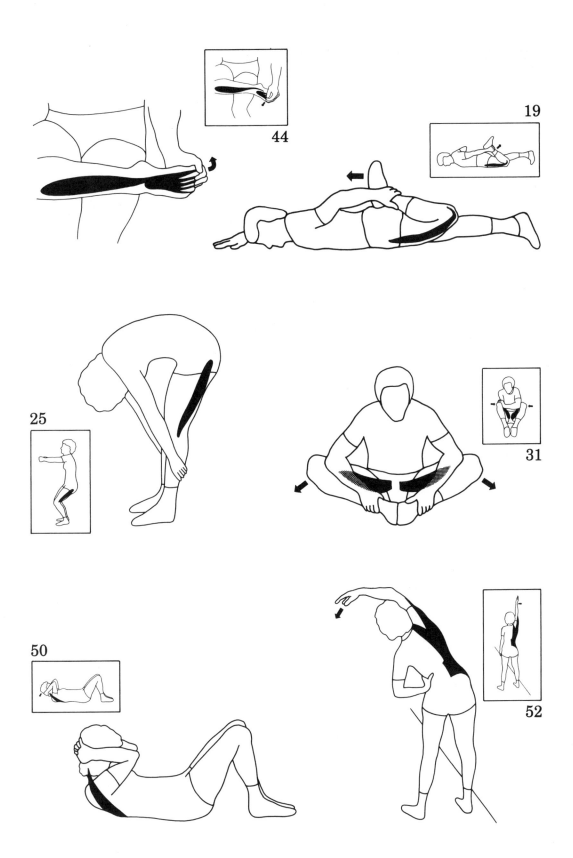

44

19

25

31

50

52

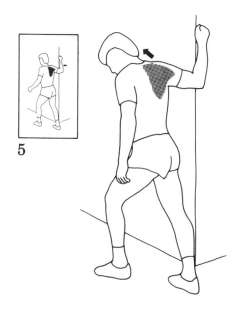

5

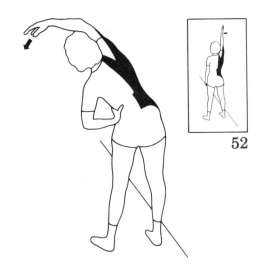

52

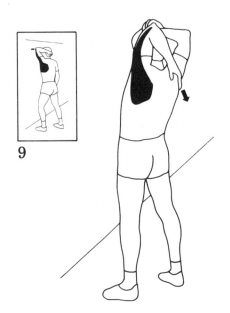

9

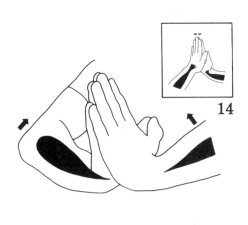

14

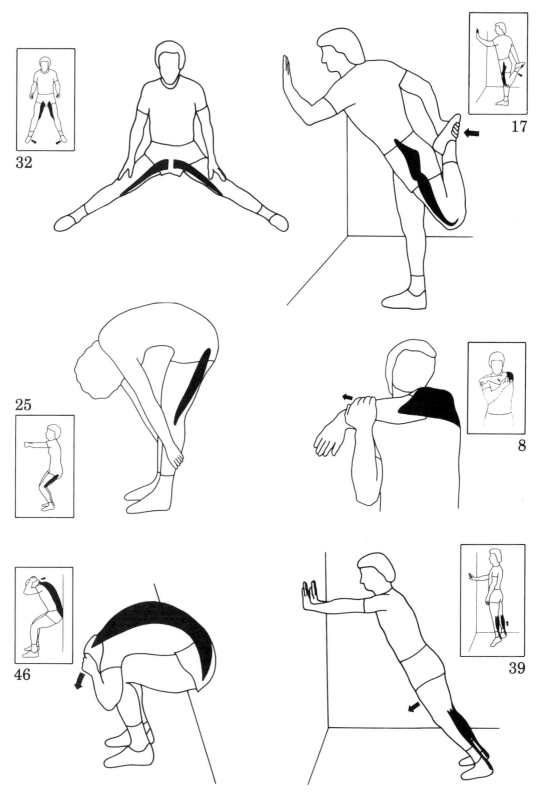

Special golf exercise: With golf club in point-of-impact position: Muscle tightening-stretch.

Weight Lifting (Body-building)

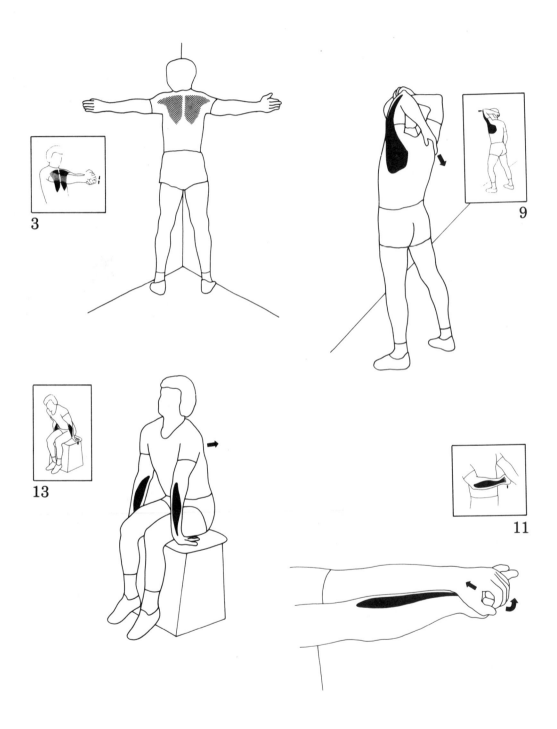

3

9

13

11

102

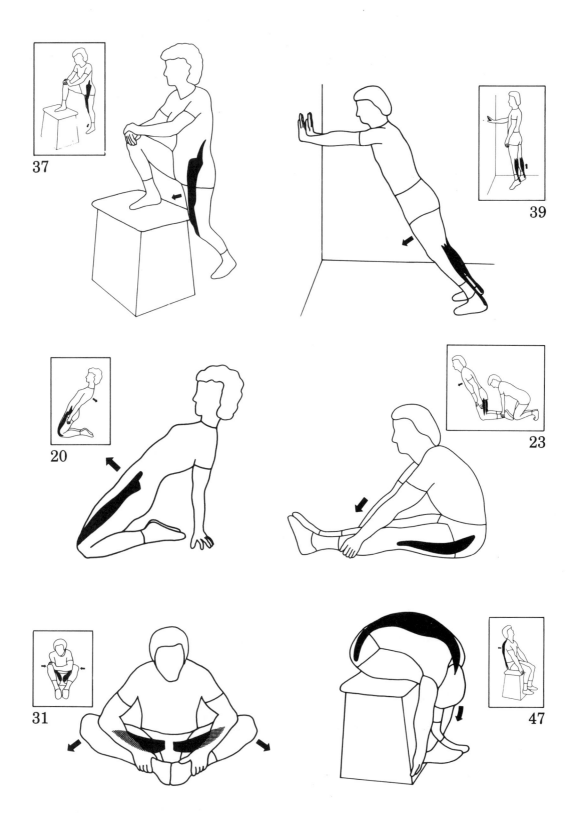

37

39

20

23

31

47

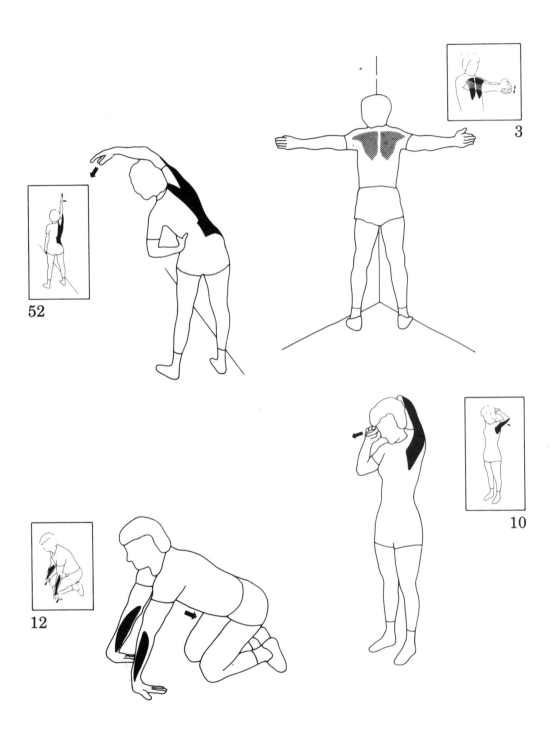

52

3

10

12

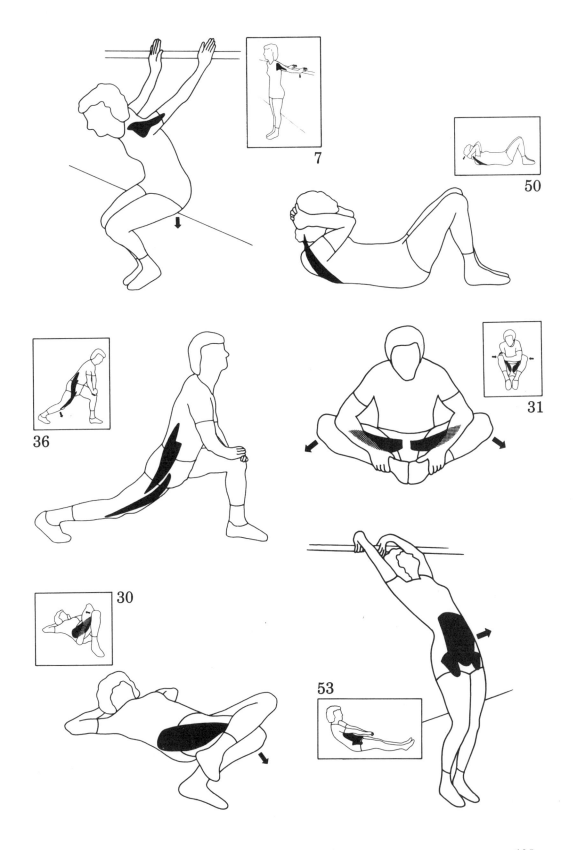

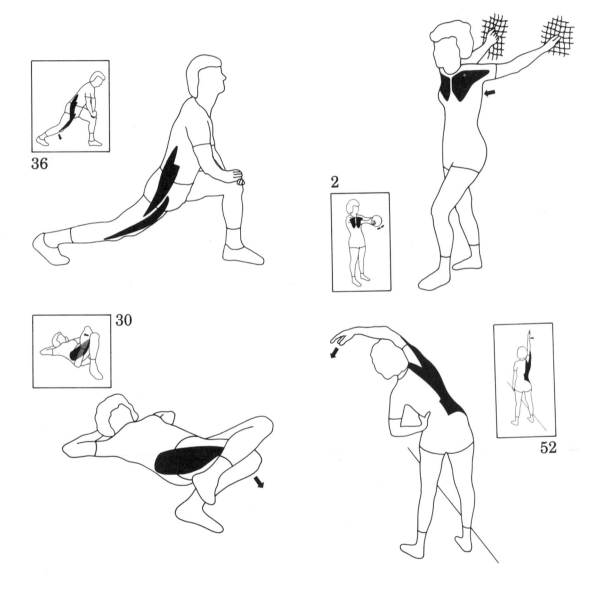

36

2

30

52

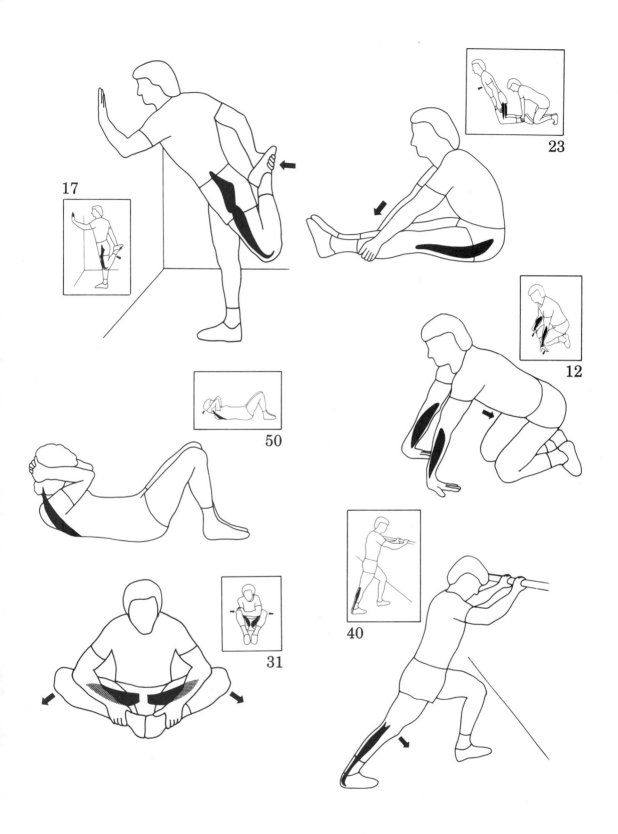

17

23

12

50

31

40

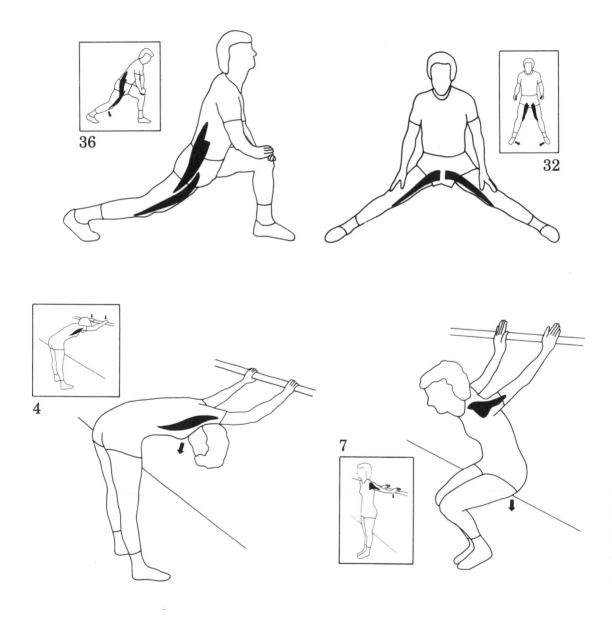

36

32

4

7

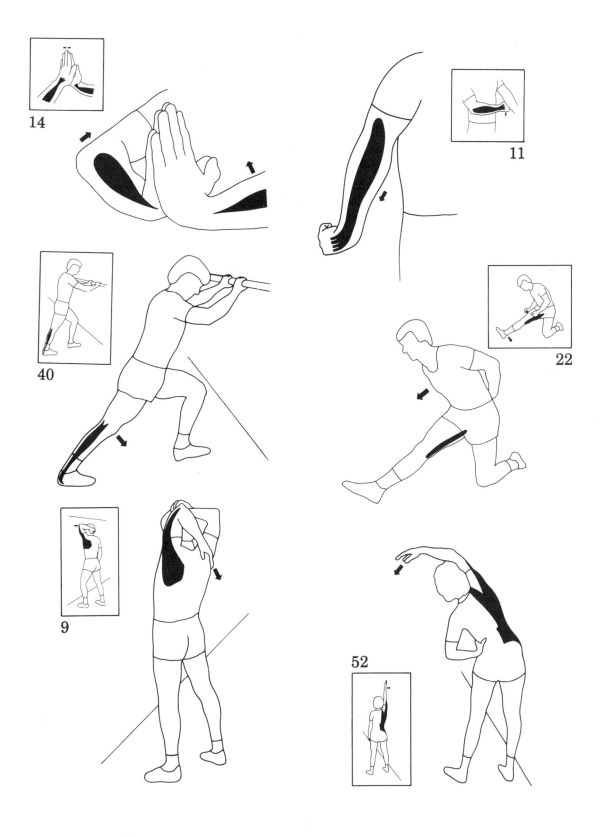

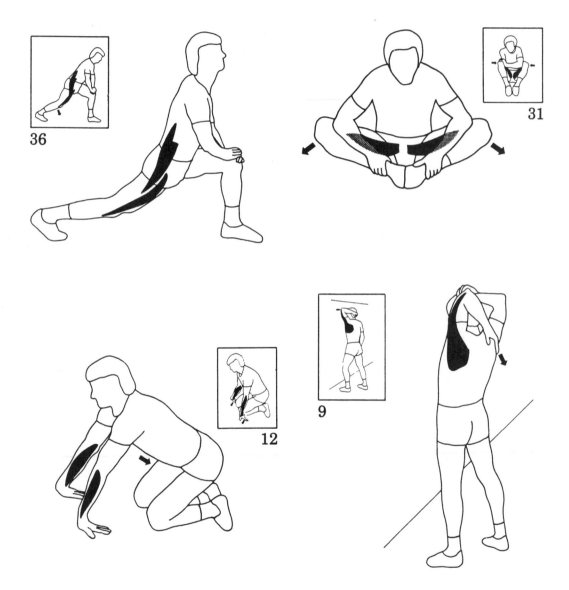

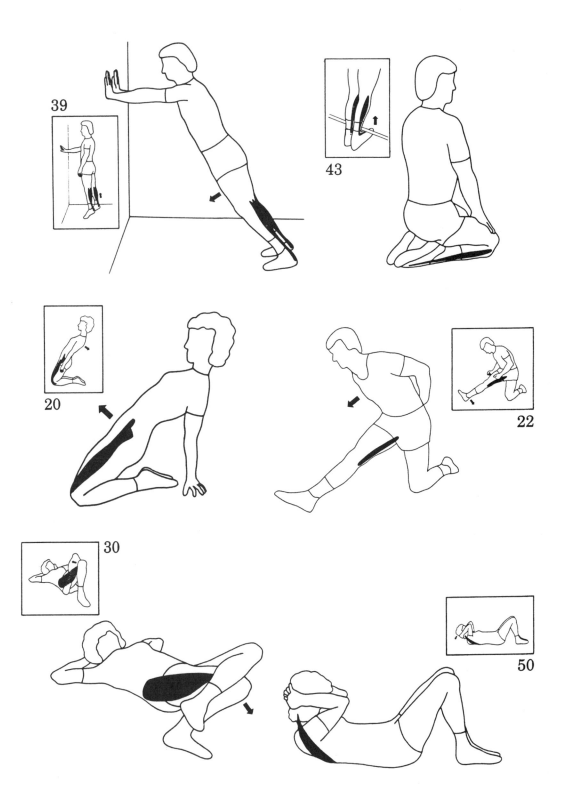

39

43

20

22

30

50

111

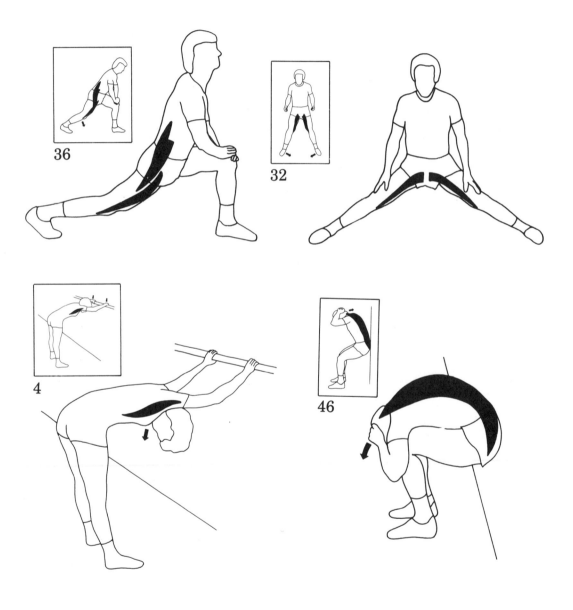

36

32

4

46

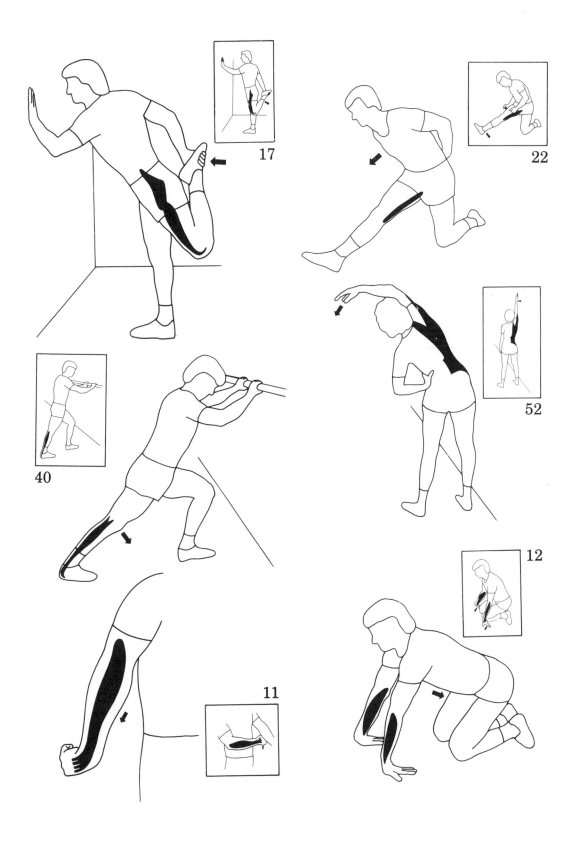

17

22

52

40

12

11

113

Stretching Prevents Injuries

It is important that the training is *both* effective and free of risk. All training, especially intensive training and also endurance training, produce shortened muscles. This is typical of pure strength training. It has even been proven that a single session of strength training diminishes flexibility as much as 5–13% over a period of at least 48 hours. Poor flexibility can cause improper stress on joints and muscles. The risk of injuries, tears and inflammation also increases considerably when the muscles are shortened and stiff. This is due to the fact that during training the durability of tendons, ligaments and bones does not increase as fast as the strength of the muscles, since these tissues have a slower metabolism than the muscles.

Muscles with a postural function (postural muscles), especially the extensor muscles, contain more of the above mentioned connective tissue structures and have a greater tendency to be shortened. Typical muscles that have a tendency to be tight are the muscles in the back of the thigh (hamstrings) and the muscles of the inside groin (adductors), the calf muscles, the big hip bending muscle (iliopsoas), the great chest muscles and the back extensor muscles.

There is a definite correlation between shortened groin muscles and the occurrence of injuries among soccer players. Among those having injuries, the flexibility of these muscles were clearly worse than the flexibility of the players who were not injured.

Injuries on tendon and muscle attachments have decreased significantly when stretching is done according to the tighten-relax-stretch method parallel with other training. Such observations and research have been made among soccer and ice hockey players (bandy players) in Sweden. In other words, it's been found that the number of injuries are obviously fewer after using the stretching method. In the U.S.A. it has also been found that stretching prevents common injuries such as Achilles-tendon inflammation and shoulder pain.

It's even possible in a typically inflammatory stage such as tennis-elbow to achieve complete relief with stretching. There are even those who have indicated a correlation between the very common sprained ankle and an unnaturally stiff set of calf muscles, when consequently calf stretching exercises would lower the risk of sprains.

The hamstring muscles are very susceptible to tears, especially in sports with a lot of sprinting such as track, handball, ice-hockey and soccer. Poor stretchability in these muscles is common among these players. Among soccer and ice-hockey players, groin problems are also very common. This is because the muscles that push the leg inward (adductors) normally are well developed and tend to be "stiff." Hockey players may get strong but shortened hip bending muscles due to the playing stance. In turn this may lead to an incorrect position of the pelvis and an increased sway in the lower back and back problems as a result.

Stretching exercises to increase flexibility become a necessity. Stretching can also be of value to prevent overuse injuries. It is important for example to prevent periostitis of the lower leg. Tibialisperiostitis affects the origin of the long toe benders at the lower two thirds of the tibia. It typically occurs when running practice is started too hard, when the intensity of the training is increased or when changing the running surface; often when switching between the outdoor and indoor seasons.

Training after Injuries

Stretching is also valuable when training to regain flexibility after an injury (or illness). It is important that the injury has totally healed prior to commencing the stretching exercises. It is essential that you don't feel any pain when stretching for rehabilitation. The physical therapists have a lot of experience with stretching exercises, for example in treating abnormal muscle shortenings and stiffness (contractures). The basic principle that is used is in accordance with the stretching method that is advocated here: after a static muscle contraction (without shortening) against resistance, relaxation and then a stretch of the muscle.

When the muscle works with resistance it is warming up. This is actually the most specific form of muscle warm-up. The stronger the muscle contraction, the higher the temperature, and in our stretching method the contraction (tightening) is always as strong as possible. This type of muscle warm-up is of great benefit and should always precede stretching of muscles. In addition, it is known that the stronger the contraction, the greater the muscle relaxation in the next phase. This is also an advantage, since the muscle should be as relaxed as possible during the stretch.

In physical therapy it has been found that stretching when the muscles are tight often gives surprisingly quick results. There are advocates of the technique of using the counteraction muscle (the antagonist) before you stretch the muscle. The reason is that you initially want to avoid putting a lot of pressure on the previously injured muscle.

Stretching Increases Performance———

It is fairly obvious that reduced flexibility will decrease performance. Good flexibility means better mechanical work conditions for the whole motor apparatus. The increased flexibility will give the muscle power more time to work, that is a longer range, which leads to a higher final speed of the motion and a better "flick."

In order to maintain his step-length during running, the world record holder and the olympic gold medal winner Sebastian Coe of Great Britain performs stretching exercises daily.

It is known that it's better to have greater flexibility for strength training. Already in 1951, H. E. Billig demonstrated that muscles that have been lightly stretched can perform stronger contractions. The stretching method with tighten-relax-stretch at the same time gives some strength training for the muscles. The technique used for muscle tightening (isometric), has been shown to be the method that develops the greatest power generation when you compare different types of muscle work.

Flexibility training also increases the metabolism in the muscles, tendons and surrounding soft tissues. This is an advantage during work periods and can also reduce the risk of aches after practice.

It has been made clear that muscle soreness (and other pain connected to physical activity) is reduced or disappears when the training includes stretching exercises. In conclusion, the incerased flexibility achieved through stretching increases performance—strength, speed and precision all are improved.

Stretching Training and Stretching———

In order to have an injury preventing effect, a fitness or training program should have a good balance between strength and stretching exercises.

Pure strength training, such as weight-training and body-building have a tendency to make the muscles short and stiff.

During 1980 and 1981 a series of studies of soccer players was made in regard to this. It was previously known that soccer players have less flexibility in their legs than people in general. (The flexibility—measured by the mobility-range of the joints—becomes worse the higher the level of play.)

The research results from strength training show that the typically shortened muscles—the groin, the front and back of the thigh, and the hip bending (flexor) muscles— have a statistically provable decrease in their mobility-range. This is even true for a single strength training session. The reduction in mobility (between five and thirteen percent) remains up to 48 hours after practice is finished.

However, when strength training was combined with subsequent stretching exercises the mobility-range was instead improved! The increase remained up to 48 hours after practice was finished.

Stretching for Groin Problems————————

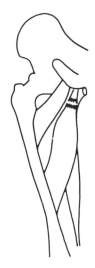

The "groin misery" in a soccer is a well known problem. While groin injuries form approximately five percent share of all athletic injuries, they form a twelve percent share of all soccer injuries.

There is a direct correlation between strong, shortened and stiff muscles and injuries due to overuse: inflammations in tendons and muscle attachments, tears, etc.

The "soccer researchers" in Linkoping, Sweden, with Dr. Jan Ekstrand leading the way, have found that the most common groin injury is either a tendon-muscle attachment inflammation or a tear in a particular groin muscle, the long inward mover (adductor longus). It was concluded that the average mobility-range of these muscles, among the ones that later were injured, were statistically provable worse than among the others. A definite correlation thus exists between shortened muscles and injuries! It is known that the stretching method (see Exercises 31–35) are particularly valuable for the flexibility of the groin muscles.

Ekstrand has also made some studies of ice hockey (bandy) teams that have used stretching exercises for groin, stomach, shoulder, and front and back thigh muscles. During the research period, not one player missed a match due to muscle or tendon problems.

The Stretch-Reflex————————

The stretch-reflex is a protective mechanism that exists in virtually all muscles; not only among the extensors but also among the flexors. Among the "benders" through the reflex is constructed somewhat differently. Examples of the stretch reflexes are the knee reflex (patella-reflex) and the Achilles (heel tendon) reflex, which is developed by hitting the tendon which is then stretched and releases the stretch-reflex. In the case of the knee reflex you get a contraction of the muscle to the tendon that connects just below the knee, the front thigh muscle. This is a common test during a physical examination. The result typically is a stretch of the knee so that the lower leg flips forward.

The stretch-reflex is developed the most in the muscles that are responsible for the erect body position, the postural muscles.

The stretch-reflex is characterized by 1) its quick response, 2) it is directly related to the strength and the speed of the stretch and 3) it stops immediately when the stretch stops. If the muscles is exposed to a continued stretch, it responds by initially doing a relatively strong contraction, which shortly decreases somewhat and then continues at a constant rate the rest of the time that the muscle is stretched.

In the "bender" muscles (flexor muscles) there is, however, only the initial quick contraction—the stretch-reflex in this case works a little differently. A stretch-reflex can also be released in the flexor muscles. (The word *Stretch Reflex* refers to the actual mechanism of activating the nerve reflex.)

The Muscle Spindles and the Stretch-Reflex

In the muscles there are sense organs, receptors, that measure the state of tightening. The most important link in the reflex system that builds the stretch-reflex (or the myotatic reflex) is the muscle spindle, which functions as both a tension meter and a length meter in the muscle. If a muscle is stretched, the muscle spindles are also stretched. Then these generate impulses to the spinal cord. A switch takes place there, synapse, and then a signal goes directly to the muscle which contracts. This is, as mentioned above, actually a protective mechanism which will prevent stretching too far so that the joint is not injured. Another thing that is typical for this reflex system is that it is very localized. It is only that muscle, even only that part of the muscle, that is exposed to the stretching that responds with a contraction.

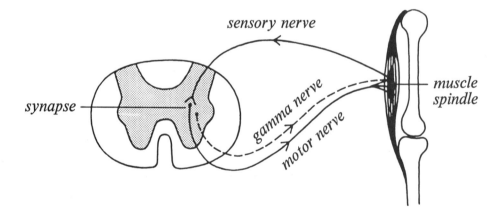

The sensitivity of the muscle spindle can be varied with the amount of nerve impulses that get to the spindle through the gamma nerve. With increasing gamma activity, the sensitivity of the muscle spindle increases. The gamma activity, which is responsible for maintaining muscle tension, tonus, increases during pain, nervousness, worry and anguish. In order to get the best effect from the stretching, as well as for all flexibility training, it is important to be relaxed and calm, or in other words to have low gamma activity.

The Golgi Tendon Organs and the Antistretch-Reflex

The Golgi tendon organs are somewhat more simply constructed. This is mainly found in the tendons at the transition area between muscle fibers and tendon fibers. In this position, the Golgi tendon organ is consequently stretched both when the muscle is actively tightened (and is shortened) and when it is passively stretched. The irritation threshold during stretching is much higher than for the muscle spindle, and therefore a much stronger stretch of the muscle tendon is required for the Golgi tendon organ to start working. An effective stimulus of the Golgi tendon organ activity exists when there is a strong muscle contraction, particularly from a static (isometric) type stretch since this has proven to produce the greatest amount of force.

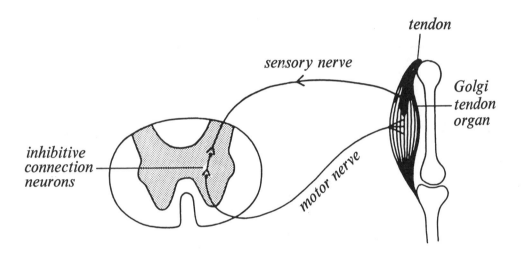

When the muscle stretch exceeds a certain critical value, the defense muscle tightening that is transmitted through the muscle spindle suddenly disappears. Instead there is a relaxation of the muscle through the influence of the Golgi tendon organs. This then protects the actual muscle and the muscle attachments against tears and extremely heavy pressure. This is called the inverse stretch-reflex, antistretch-reflex or antimyotatic reflex. All of this mechanism under influence of the Golgi tendon organs is also called autogenetic inhibition, "self-inhibition," since it inhibits the muscle contraction.

Methods to Inhibit the Stretch-Reflex——

In order to be able to carry on effective and correct flexibility training, you must inhibit the stretch-reflex. If it is activated during stretching you will have risk of injuries of the muscle fibers and the opposite effect from what was intended.

The training methods in which you avoid the stretch-reflex can be summarized under the concept "stretching." Included in this concept are generally three procedures; tighten-stretch, partially according to the methodology of autogenic-inhibition, partially the counteraction method and thirdly passive "slow-stretch."

1.   Muscle Tightening with Self-inhibition——

This method involves a (preferably passive) stretch of a group of muscles that just before has been tightened as much as possible statically. Through that the inhibiting influence of the Golgi tendon organs on the stretch-reflex leads to relaxation of the muscle (autogenetic inhibition).

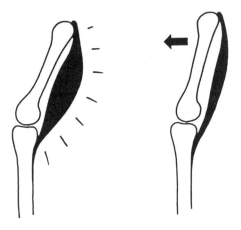

During such a forceful stretch of the muscle-tendon where the threshold of the Golgi tendon organ reaction is exceeded, there is then an impulse flow from the tendon organs through the nerve fibers into the spinal cord. Here there is a switch to inhibiting connection nerve cells and from these there are fibers out to the muscle again. These impulses have the opposite effect to the muscle spindles. The stretch-reflex is inhibited and the muscle is relaxed. The tendon organs require, due to (as we discussed before) a higher threshold value, a more forceful stretch of the muscle or muscle contraction with stretching of the muscle tendon than do the muscle spindles. The more forceful the contraction the greater the relaxation in the muscle. The strongest muscle tension is created through static (isometric)

muscle tightening. It has been shown that there is a remaining effect from the self-inhibition, so that the muscle remains relaxed for a while after a strong muscle contraction, post-contractive inhibition. It is this relaxation that is used during the following stretch and you therefore achieve a better effect from the stretch. It is considered an advantage if the muscle has been stretched (passively) in the direction of the stretch from the beginning, in other words, prior to the start of the isometric muscle tightening.

2. Muscle Tightening-Stretching with the Counteraction Method

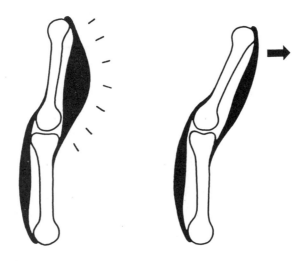

If you tighten a muscle, there is at the same time a relaxation of the counteracting muscle on a reflex basis. This is a natural prerequisite for a movement in a joint. This relaxation of the opposite working muscles (antagonists) is called *Reciprocal Inhibition* and occurs through inhibiting connections from the muscle spindles in the tightened muscles via the spinal cord to the antagonists. The relaxation in the opposing muscles becomes greater the stronger the muscle tightening is. The reflex induced relaxed group of counteracting muscles is in this way more available for stretching, which can be used in the training program. However, this method is not so generally usable as the previous one, since when tightening certain groups of muscles, for example, the "benders" of the fingers and the wrist, the counteracting muscles (corresponding extensors) are also tightened in order to stabilize the joint. Relaxation of the counteracting muscles can then not be used for stretching training.

3. Passive Stretching of the Muscle (Slow Stretching)

The plain stretch, which can be said to be included as the second portion of the two previous methods, is the original form of static stretching in athletics. It means that after stretching out the muscles, you stay in the outmost position. You divide the stretch into two portions, in the first of which the so called easy stretch, you stop in the outside position 10–30 seconds. You will be able to feel how the tightening is reduced as the muscles have time to reach the greatest length. After this comes the second portion, the development stretch, in which you stretch a little further and stay in this position also for 10–30 seconds. If the tightening feeling is increased during the stretch a over-stretch, drastic stretch is taking place. This is not good and creates a risk of injuries. The easy and the development stretch doesn't activate the stretch-reflex and doesn't cause pain. All the exercises in this book obviously contain a stretch portion. This portion could be performed separately from the muscle tightening portion according to the description above. As always, it would be important that all the moves are done in a controlled manner without sudden parts and with a relaxed body and spirit.

The Stretchability in the Connective Tissue

In order to evaluate the time factor during the execution of the stretch portions, it is necessary to take into account the yielding (giving) of the connective tissue. The most outstanding flexibility limiting factors are partially the activity of your reflex system and partially the stiffness of the connective tissue. It is primarily the connective tissue of the muscles that inhibits your movements through its length and extendability. In soft tissue, the connective tissue gives stability and transmits power, and so connective tissue "paths" go through the muscles and form the power transmitting tendons.

The connective tissue consists of three components, of which one, built from the collagen fibers, is the most important from a automechanical standpoint. A tendon consists of up to 90 percent of collagen fibers, arranged so that they can resist pulling loads to the greatest possible extent. During muscle tightening, one tendon only gets between 25 and 30 percent of its maximum tenacity load. Among all the different parts of the mobility apparatus, the tendon nor the ligament is almost never the weakest link during a mechanical load. Tears most often occur in the bone attachment, sometimes in the muscle or in the connection between muscle-tendon.

It is known that the muscle tissue, if relaxed, can be stretched to double length and return to the normal state without sustaining any critical injury. This flexibility doesn't exist in the connective tissue of the tendons and the muscle sheaths. Therefore, this is the main object of the flexibility training.

The load speed is of importance to the collagen fibers. The flexibility and elasticity are decreased with increased velocity in loading. Therefore, note that the stretchable and formable characteristics increase during a slow load. It is also clear that the yielding capacity increases with the time that a tendon is exposed to a certain amount of tension, which is typically called the "creeping" phenomena. During repeated stretching with the same load, a ceiling level is soon reached. In order to change the formability of the connective tissue, it has been shown that the stretch is at least 6–10 seconds long while the muscle at the same time has a low tonus (self-tension), i.e., low gamma activity. It is also known that the stretchability of the collagen fibers increases with temperatures over 39 degrees C.

Static, Dynamic and PNF-Stretching——

In the U.S.A. one speaks of two traditional styles of stretching, static and dynamic. The static method consists of a slow continuous extension of the group of muscles and the joint complex until an ultimate position is reached and keeping that position for 5–10 seconds.

This type works the same way as the earlier mentioned "slow-stretch" and has proven to be an effective method to improve flexibility. The dynamic method has a fast, bouncing start (ballistic) and is considered less effective.

Later a third method, the PNF technique was developed to increase the mobility-range. L. E. Holt developed a method based on this technique in 1971. The Holt method was called Scientific Stretching for Sport (3S). This procedure consists of first stretching the muscles, followed by a static (isometric) tightening for six seconds. Then it continues with a concentric contraction of the counteracting muscles of the joint at the same time as a practice partner applies light pressure. This interchanging isometric and concentric muscle tightening continues until a greater mobility-range cannot be obtained. Holt's 3S method was accepted as helping to improve mobility, but in reality often caused confusion about how to do it, due to the difficulty in teaching it.

The Six American Stretching Methods—

There have been many stretching methods introduced, but few have been studied thoroughly. Based on the premises that there are two basic ways to improve flexibility, 1) to decrease the resistance of the connective tissue surrounding the joint through stretching and inhibition of the stretch-reflex and 2) to increase the strength of the counteracting muscles, there have been six stretching methods formalized in the U.S.A.

These were studied in 1976 (Hartley and Russel) and were all found to be beneficial for flexibility (of the hip joint that was tested) so that there was an extension of the soft tissue.

In the U.S.A. it has since then been considered wise to stress passive PNF-technique and sometimes active PNF. The relaxation method is recommended as an effective model to overcome physical and psychological tension.

1. Ballistic and Hold. Here you start with a swing, bounce or a couple of rocking motions. On the third or fourth swing you keep the limb in the outmost position through your own force approximately six seconds each time.

2. Passive Lift and Hold. A practice partner moves the joint passively to its outmost position. This position is kept by tightening the muscles statically for six seconds. Such passive pulling and active holding is alternated in six seconds intervals for one minute.

3. Prolonged Stretch. This is strictly a passive stretch done with the help of a practice partner who extends the mobility-range gradually to the outmost position. You stay there just below the pain threshold for approximately one minute.

4. Active PNF. The motion is extended as far as possible through active muscle work for six seconds. Then a maximum isometric muscle tightening of the counteracting muscles is done with resistance for example from a practice partner. After this, you try to get still further through active muscle work and interchange this with tightening of the counteracting muscle with resistance in six seconds intervals for one minute.

5. Passive PNF. The joint is passively moved to the outmost position with the help of a practice partner within six seconds, after which, as in the previous method, you perform an isometric muscle tightening of the counteracting muscles through resistance from your partner. The passive stretch is interchanged with counteracting muscle tightening, also in six seconds intervals for one minute.

6. Relaxation Method. A slow stretch is done passively to the outmost position by participation of a practice partner. There you keep the stretch for one minute while the performer relaxes mentally through self-control. By becoming aware of the state of the tightening in the muscle you help to inhibit the muscle reflex.

The Time Factors in Stretching————————

Regarding the stretching method described in this book, it has not been sure what length of time should be used for the first two parts: the tightening of the muscle (maximum tension) and the relaxation before the stretch. However, it is known that the stretch must be kept for at least 6–10 seconds (varying information in different research papers) in order for the connecting tissue in the tendon-muscle complex and joint capsule to be reshaped.

The Linkoping group has used the following intervals:

Tighten the muscle for 4–6 seconds, relax for 2 seconds and stretch 8 seconds with 4–6 repetitions consecutive. For a 15-minute program for six groups of muscles in the legs, they found at the following measurement which followed a 5–12 percent increase of the mobility-range still existed ½, 1 and 1½ hours after the stretch!

The long-term effect of stretching was also studied in 90 soccer players, who had a stretching program added to their regular team practice 3–4 times per week. Players with shortened muscles also received a program for individual stretching. The mobility-range was measured after two and after six weeks. Both groups showed an increase in flexibility of all the muscle groups that were exercised. In a control group of soccer players that did not do any stretching exercises, they found a decrease in flexibility. The soccer researchers have consequently seen a lasting long time result for both individual and team stretching.

As a conclusion of these two studies, it can be said that the stretching effect of a single training session remains at least 1½ hours and that team stretching is enough to increase the flexibility. In a report from GIH Stockholm in 1979, they have shown that the contract-relax stretching method using intervals of 7 seconds-2 seconds-7 seconds are clearly superior to the traditional bounce-stretch exercises. It was found that the greatest increase in flexbility took place during the first two weeks. Practicing once a week gave clearly worse results than three and five times per week respectively. However, the differences were small between the two latter practice frequencies, which made them recommend three times per week. The inhibition from the tension in the muscle itself, which in this method is reached through the initial maximum static muscle tightening, so called post-contractory inhibition and which is used later for an effective stretch, can be explained to be due to the self-inhibition (autogenetic inhibition). This takes place through the inhibiting effect of the Golgi tendon organs during maximum tightening of the muscles. Because of that, we would like to make the muscle tightening part continue a while, for example 15–30 seconds, so that you make sure that it really reaches the maximum possible. This additional amount of time also benefits the warming effect of the muscle tightening. However, there are those who maintain that the self-inhibiting mechanism cannot explain the aforementioned muscle inhibition after the tightening since the self-inhibition is considered to allow too short a time period to use the stretch.

The pioneer of stretching in the U.S.A., Bob Anderson, maintains that you can't activate the stretch-reflex with just the stretch portion (without prior muscle tightening), presupposed that the movements are gentle and without a bounce or a rocking motion. According to this method, you first do an easy stretch for 10–30 seconds with a mild stretch. You will then find that the tension decreases during the time you hold the position. Then you continue with the development stretch in which you are stretching further (without noticing any pain) and keep that position also for 10–30 seconds. In the U.S.A. it has been found that this method shows a clear decrease in muscle soreness with physical activity.

Of the six American methods for stretching mentioned earlier, the prolonged stretch is listed with a holding time of one minute and generally for static stretching a 5–10 seconds holding time. In this U.S.A. group the PNF exercises show an isometric (static) tightening time of six seconds as well as for the counteraction group of muscles. The same time, six seconds, is also true for tightening of the holding time of either a passive or an active stretch. In the methods in which you alternate tightening with stretching, the intervals are repeated for one minute.

Some Historical Observations————

Muscle tightening during gymnastics have been done from time immemorial. There are statues 2,000 years old from Bangkok that show people in positions for stretching exercises. The specific stretching patterns that exist have their origin in certain movements of the Indian yoga. In old Chinese and Indian documents are descriptions of a type of gymnastics that show close similarity to the physical therapy of today. In modern physical therapy they have for a long time realized the advantages of a continued slow stretch to overcome shortened muscles and restore mobility in the joints.

In recent years, neurophysiologists have developed methods to improve the mobility-range of different joints. A pioneer in this field is Kabat, whose technique was called PNF (Proprioceptive Neuromusclular Facility Treatment). In this you treat muscular overtension with a contract-relax method, in other words tighten-relax method similar to the method advocated in this book. This PNF method was made popular by M. Knott and D. Voss and was used by physiotherapists. It was adapted by L. E. Holt in 1971 as a stretching method for athletes.

The American gymnastic pedagogue Robert "Bob" Anderson has since then spread the slow-stretch method, and even with the modification tighten-relax-stretch according to the reciprocal inhibition method. One of the pioneers in Sweden is Dr. Jan Ekstrand, who has done a series of fine studies of stretching usage.

Scientific Studies about Stretching———

Just as in athletics in general, there are surprisingly few scientific studies done to find out the effects of stretching.

The Danes, E. Assmussen and M. Nielsen, indicated in 1967 that bounce-stretching at too fast a speed leads to activation of the stretch-reflex so that the muscle contracts and the flexibility training is counteracted. Knott and Voss in the U.S.A. (1968) and Jungwirth and Myrenberg (1973) in Sweden have described and researched the technique of tighten-relax-stretch that is the basis for the stretching method recommended in this book. M. C. Tanigawa in California in 1972 compared PNF-technique (hold-relax) and passive mobilizing, and found that a faster and greater increase of the mobility-range was achieved with the PNF-technique. Russel and Hartley have separately researched six American stretching methods, both with and without the PNF-technique. In articles published in 1977 and 1978, Jan Ekstrand, Sweden, has described a noticeable decrease in the number of injuries of muscles and muscle attachments of players on soccer and ice hockey teams on an elite level when using stretching.

A very enlightening Swedish study was published in 1979 by R. Grahn and T. Nordenborg at the GIH (College of Gymnastics and Athletics) in a report on flexibility training with Wallin and Nystrom as superintendents. It was clearly shown that the active tightening—passive stretching method is superior to traditional bounce-stretching methods to improve flexibility.

The "soccer researchers" in Linkoping, Sweden, led by Jan Ekstrand, have in 1981 shown that stretching gives an increase of the mobility-range of 5–12% that remains for at least 90 minutes. It has also been found that a pure strength training session decreases the mobility range by 5–13%, while a combination including a stretching session even gave an increase in flexibility that remained even after 48 hours. This research group has also discovered a definite correlation between shortened groin muscles (adductors) and injuries in these muscles. For further information refer to the bibliography at the end of the book.

In his 1982 dissertation, Ekstrand maintains that the reason for muscle stiffness among the soccer players (67% had one or more leg muscles tighter than non-players) seems to be tied to the type of training program. After introducing an injury prevention program where stretching was one of the main ingredients, the number of injuries decreased by 75% (23 injuries vs 93) for six test soccer clubs in a Swedish division IV league (local amateur soccer league) and where six other teams made up the control group (using bounce-stretching). During warm-up the test teams used 10 minutes of stretching and during cool-down (down-training) 5 minutes. This increased the mobility-range of the players by 5–20% and was mainly considered the cause for four times as many muscle strains in the control teams as in the test teams (23 vs 6). Both the Linkoping group and Jones (1977) have found that even long distance runners have very poor mobility.

When comparing two PNF-techniques regarding hip-bending, Markos (1979) found that the mobility increase was greater if the contraction segment was at maximum for a full 9 seconds interval (contract-relax CR) than if it was gradually increased during the same amount of time (hold-relax HR) with both techniques using active "straight leg-raising." Moore and Hutton (1980) showed in a similar manner, when studying three different techniques of hip-bending, that the CRAC method (Contract-Relax-Agonist-Contraction), in other words isometric maximum hamstring contraction (5 seconds) followed by relaxation and then a hamstring stretch (9 seconds) simultaneously with a less than maximum contraction of the hip-bending muscles, gave the greatest increase in mobility (i.e., same as Exercise 24 in this book if during the stretch you also try to actively lift the straight leg further up). The other two methods in this study were contract-relax, (muscle tightening-relaxation-stretch) and pure static stretching. A poor relation was also shown between EMG (electric muscle activity) and mobility increase (CRAC paradoxically gave higher hamstring EMG). Lewit (1981) has indicated a definite muscle inhibition and considerable pain reducing effects on "pain-points" in tendon and muscle connectors on the periosteum by the method of isometric resistance (10 seconds) followed by relaxation and stretch with therapeutical effects on the majority of 220 persons included in the study. Sady (1982) has compared three different methods of mobility training for shoulders, back and hamstrings. The PNF method with muscle tightening and stretch in 6 seconds intervals was shown preferable (gave 10% mobility increase) over strictly static stretching (6 seconds) or bounce-stretching (20 bounce-stretches) with three training sessions per week during six weeks. The best result was achieved with the hamstring muscles. Earlier L. E. Holt, T. M. Travis and T. Okita (1970) and M. C. Tanigawa (1972) also found the PNF-technique to be the best.

• Children and Stretching

Many individuals need to improve their mobility but of course not every one. An example is children under 10 or so or in prepuberty who already by nature have good mobility. Stretching exercises are therefore unnecessary unless they are heavily involved in sports, have some mobility restricting disease or are rehabilitating after an injury. However, it is clearly advisable to *teach* stretching as a conscious mobility training method for future use. (It has been noticed that stretching has had good effect on "growing pains" in the lower legs.)

• Positive for Elderly

Even adults with an acceptable mobility-range can benefit from stretching through the positive effects of increased blood circulation in the muscles, improved metabolism, reduced stiffness and tenderness after exercise, general reduction of tension and feeling of well being. Stretching therefore can be said to vitalize the muscles, maintain youth, and in connection with a rapidly increasing mobility is this probably the reason for the popularity this stretching method actually has had among elderly, particularly those with stiffness and soreness problems in joints, tendons and muscles. Stretching in addition can be done without any "basic training," condition or fitness without special clothing, equipment and other facilities.

● *The First Standard Warm-Up*

Note that stretching should never replace regular circulation warm-up. The stretching complements the warm-up in the work-out, which actually in any training circumstance should have the following major parts and principal construction:

1. Warm-up for heart and lungs, preferably to a pulse over 100 per minute giving an increase of the muscle temperature, which is favorable to stretching.
2. Stretching, preferably one set per group of muscles shown in the Basic Program (see pages 77–113) possibly mixed with Exercises from pages 23–75.
3. Special training: Conditioning, strength, speed, technique, and coordination.
4. "Down-training" ("cool-down" or "warm-down") with three phases:
   a. Gradual intensity decrease, "down jogging"
   b. Stretching, main program with three sets per muscle
   c. Mental relaxation exercises

● *Psychological Relaxation*

Stretching, which should be done with a conscious voluntary relaxation of the rest of the body, gives in itself a muscle relaxation which aids in psychological relaxation. You can therefore use stretching in the treatment of nervous related tension states such as stiff neck tension headache (sometimes so that nerve relaxing medication could be discontinued). Stretching eases tension and lowers the "tonus" of the body (muscle tension level) and you get a significant and characteristic lowering of the electrical muscle activity EMG (De Vries, 1966).

● *As Treatment*

Pain has however been proven to give increased muscle activity as far as EMG goes and a definite tendency for muscle tension that can cause shortening of muscles. If you feel pain either before, during or after stretching, you have done something incorrectly! However, in the U.S.A. stretching is being used as treatment for inflamed tendons and muscles, but in Sweden, we do not want to recommend this since there has not been enough research in this area. De Vries in the U.S.A. found in 1966 that static stretching gave considerable improvement in 20 out of 23 cases with muscle pains such as shinsplints (lower leg), sore forearm muscles, pain in thigh muscles (front and back) as well as outside thigh/hip and calf. Even in Sweden, in some places stretching has been used with good results using professional advice with pain conditions behind the kneecap (*patellalgi*, "*chondromalacia patellae*"—common among young people), shoulder pain and even "tennis-elbow" (pains at the connecting point of the extensor muscles of the wrist in the forearm). The prompt relief from calf cramps received through static stretching is old and well known (Morris, Gasteiger and Chatfield, 1957).

• Against Sore Muscles

Glick (1980) indicates that both muscle problem of Type II (soreness or cramps during or immediately following heavy exercise) and Type III (1–2 days following heavy exercise—"exercise ache") are counteracted by stretching which gives reduced pain. If stretching is used for preventive purposes, it can almost be guaranteed that "exercise ache" (soreness) does not occur or occurs at a bearable level after other exercise. On the contrary, when stretching you get a feeling of well-being most often after the work-out.

• For Low Back Pain

Stretching can have some effect against back problems. Several stretching exercises are good to prevent or reduce lower back problems, specially exercises for the hip-bending (*iliopsoas*) and the hamstring muscles. Already in 1949, Kraus found a correlation through 71 % of people with lower back problems having shortened back/hamstring/gastrosoleus muscle complex (and of these 41 % had shortened hamstrings). It is considered that the muscles follow a physiological law in which muscles kept in shortened position during long periods of time will lead to permanent stiffness. So, the sitting position should give shortened iliopsoas and hamstrings. By counteracting the shortening of the muscles, stretching exercises put the lower back and the pelvis in a more natural position. However, it is not recommended to stretch the back muscles during acute problems of the back such as sciatic radiating pain.

Bibliography

Abrahams, M., "Mechanical behavior of tendons in vitro." *Med. Biol. Engng. 5, 1967.*

Anderson, Bob., *Stretching.* Shelter Publications, Calif. 1980.

Balaskas, A. & Stirk, J., *Soft Exercise—The Complete Book of Stretching.* Unwin paperbacks, London 1983.

Billig, H. E., *The Significance of Mobility.* Scholastic Coach, USA. 1951.

DeVries, H., *Physiology of Exercise for Physical Education and Athletics.* W. C. Brown, Dubuque, Iowa, 1980.

DeVries, H., "Evaluation of static stretching procedures for improvement of flexibility." *Research Quarterly 33, 1962.*

DeVries, H., "Quantitative electromyographic investigation of the spasm theory of muscle pain." *American Journal of Physical Medicine 45/1966.*

Ekstrand, J., "Soccer injuries and their prevention." *Medical Dissertation, No. 130, 1982,* Linkoping, Sweden.

Ekstrand, J. & Gillquist, J., "The frequency of muscle tightness and injuries in soccer players." *Am. J. Sports Med. 10, 1982.*

Elliot, D., "The biomechanical properties of tendon in relation to muscular strength." *Ann. Phys. Med. 9, 1967.*

Ganong, W. F., *Review of Medical Physiology.* Lange Medical Publ. 1973.

Glick, J., "Muscle Strains: Prevention & Treatment." *The Physician & Sportmedicine Vol. 8, 1980.*

Grahn, R. & Nordenborg, Th., "Flexibility Training—Comparative study of two methods." *GIH Report,* Stockholm 1979.

Hartley, S., "A comparison of six methods of stretch on active range of hip flexion." *Masters thesis,* University of British Columbia, Canada, 1976.

Hogg, J. M., "Flexibility training: It's importance for the competitive swimmer." *Katimavik,* University of Alberta, Vol. 5, No. 1, 1978.

Holt, L. E., *Scientific stretching for sport (3S).* Stencil Dalhousis University, Halifax, Nova Scotis, 1971.

Holt, L. E., Travis, T. M. & Okita, T. "A comparative study of three stretching techniques." *Perpetual Motor Skills, 31, 1970.*

Jones, Arthur., "Flexibility as a result of exercises." *Athletic Journal, March 1977.*

Kabat & Knott, "Propriceptive facilitation techniques for treatment of paralysis." *Physical Therapy Review 33, No. 2, 1953.*

Kaltenborn, F., *Manual therapy for the extremity joints.* Norlis Forlag, Oslo, Norway, 1974.

Knott, M. & Voss, D., "Patterns of motion for proprioceptive neuromuscular facilitation." *Br. J. Phys. Med. 17, 1954.*

Knott, M. & Voss, D., *Proprioceptive Neuromuscular Facilitation. Harper & Row*, New York, 1968.

Kottke, F., Pauley, D., Ptak, R. "The rationale for prolonged stretching for the correction of shortening of connective tissue." *Arch. Phys. Med. Rehab. 196, 1966.*

Lewit, K., *Muskelfazilitation- und Inhibitionstechniken in der Manuellen Medizin.* Manuelle Medizin, Prag, 1981.

Little, R. & Haut, R., "A constitutive equation for collagen fibers." *Journ. of Biomechanics 5/1972.*

Little, R. & Jenkins, R., "A constitutive equation for parallel-fibered elastic tissue." *Journ. of Biomechanics 7/1972.*

Markos, P. D., "Ipsilateral and Contralateral effects of Proprioceptive Neuromuscular Facilitation Techniques on Hip motion and Electromyographic Activity." *Physical Therapy 1979.*

Moore, M. & Hutton, R., "Electromyographic investigation of muscle stretching techniques." *Medicine and Science Sports 12, 1980.*

Möller, M., "Athletic training and flexibility." *Medical Dissertation No. 182*, Linkoping University, Sweden, 1984.

O'Donoghue, D., *Treatment of Injuries to Athletes.* Saunders, Philadelphia-London-Toronto 1976.

Roy, S. & Irvin, R., *Sports Medicine, prevention, evaluation . . . .* Prentice-Hall, Inc., New Jersey, 1983.

Sady, S., Wortman, M., Blanke, D., "Flexibility training: Ballistic, static or proprioceptive neuromuscular facilitation." *Arch. Phys. Med. Rehabil. 63, 1982.*

Smith, J., Hutton, R., Eldred, E., "Postcontraction changes in sensitivity of muscle afferents to static and dynamic stretch." *Brain Research 78, 1974.*

Tanigawa, M. C., "Comparison of Hold-Relax procedure and passive mobilization on increasing muscle length." *Physical Therapy Vol. 52, 1972.*

Uram, Paul, *The Complete Stretching Book.* Anderson World, Inc., Calif., USA, 3rd, 1981.

Viidik, A., "On the correlation between structure and mechanical function of soft connective tissues." *Verh. Anat. Ges. 72, 1978.*

Weber, S. & Kraus, H., "Passive and active stretching for muscles." *Physical Therapy Review 29, 1949.*

Weaver, N., *Runner's World Stretching Book.* Runner's worlds Books, California 1982.

Wright, V. & Johns, R., "Physical factors concerned with stiffness of normal and deseased joints." *Bulletin of Johns-Hopkins Hospital, 1960.*

Wright, V., "Stiffness: A review of its measurement and physiological importance." *Physiotherapy 59, 1973.*

Index

muscle spindle, 118, 120, 121
    strength, 16
    tear, 15
muscle-tendon crossing, 15
    level, 129
muscle warm-up, 115
MTP, 67
myotatic reflex, 118

nerve reflex, 19, 118
nervous related tension, 129
Nielsen, M., 127
Nordenborg, T., 127

Okita, T., 128
overuse injury, 115

passive "slow-stretch", 120
    stretching method, 127
patella-reflex, 117
patellalgi, 129
performance, 116
periostitis, 115
physical tension, 124
PIP, 67
PNF (Proprioceptive Neuromusclular Facility Treatment), 126
    exercise, 126
    method, 128
    technique, 123, 124, 127
precision, 116
prepuberty, 128
prevent injury, 17
psychological relaxation, 14,
  129
    tension, 124
pulls in muscles and tendon,
  15
pure static stretching, 128

reciprocal inhibition, 121
    method, 126
rehabilitation, 115
relaxation, 115, 121, 125
resistance, 115
running, 13, 20

scientific stretching for
  sport(3S), 123
secretary stretch, 52
self-inhibition, 119, 121, 125
    mechanism, 125
self-tension, 123
sensory nerve, 118, 119
shoulder rotation, 20
side-bend, 20
side-step, 16, 18
simple effective method, 11
sit-up, 20
skip rope, 16
slalom position, 47
slow-stretch, 123
    method, 126
speed, 18, 116
sprain, 114
    in muscles and
    tendon, 15
stamina, 17, 18
static/isometric muscle
  tension, 14
    muscle contraction, 115
    rowing, 69
stiff neck, 129
stiffness, 115
strength, 13, 17, 116
    training, 17, 114, 116
strengthening exercise, 20, 128
stretch, 16
    portion, 122, 125
stretch-reflex, 19, 117, 120

stretcher, 33, 68, 117
    Extensor, 66
    layer, 70
    muscle, 114
stretching, 13, 17, 115, 120
    exercise, 115, 116
    method, 114–117, 125
swim motion, 20
synapse, 118

tailor stretch, 53
Tanigawa, M.C., 127, 128
tear, 114, 122
tendon, 15, 116, 119, 121
    attachment, 15
    -muscle attachment
   inflammation, 117
tennis-elbow, 114
tibialisperiostitis, 115
tighten-relax method, 126
    -stretch, 116, 126
    -stretch method, 13,
  15, 114
tighten-stretch, 120
tonus, 118, 123, 129
traditional bounce-stretch
  exercises, 125
Travis, T.M., 128

Voss, D., 126
Vries, De, 129

waist rotation, 20
war-dance, 16
warm-up, 129
weight lifting, 13
weight-training, 116
work-out, 129